REVERSING POLYCYSTIC KIDNEY DISEASE

The PKDproof program:
a low-carb, high-nutrient
approach to kidney health

FELIX MUELLER

WITH A FOREWORD BY DAVE ASPREY

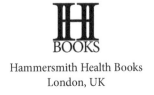

Hammersmith Health Books
London, UK

First published in 2024 by Hammersmith Health Books
– an imprint of Hammersmith Books Limited
4/4A Bloomsbury Square, London WC1A 2RP, UK
www.hammersmithbooks.co.uk

Disclaimer: This book is designed to provide helpful information on the
subjects discussed. It is not meant to be used, nor should it be used, to diagnose
or treat any medical condition. For diagnosis or treatment of any medical
problem, consult your own physician or healthcare provider. The publisher
and author are not responsible for any specific health or allergy needs that may
require medical supervision and are not liable for any damages or negative
consequences from any treatment, action, application or preparation, to any
person reading or following the information in this book. References are
provided for informational purposes only and do not constitute endorsement of
any websites or other sources. Readers should be aware that the websites listed
in this book may change. The information and references included are up to
date at the time of writing but given that medical evidence progresses, it may
not be up to date at the time of reading.

British Library Cataloguing in Publication Data: A CIP record of this book is
available from the British Library.

Print ISBN 978-1-78161-247-7
Ebook ISBN 978-1-78161-246-0

Commissioning editor: Georgina Bentliff
Designed and typeset by: Julie Bennett of Bespoke Publishing Ltd
Cover design by: Madeline Meckiffe
Cover images: © Shutterstock/35lab/Svetla/ST.art
Index by: Dr Laurence Errington
Production: Angela Young
Printed and bound by: TJ Books, Cornwall, UK

Contents

Contents

Contents

Foreword

In my quest to explore the limits of human performance and health, I've encountered many stories that challenge conventional wisdom. My journey began with my overcoming fatigue, brain fog and a 300-pound body. This quest led me down an uncharted path, where I experimented with everything from all the diets to cutting-edge technology, spending over two million dollars on biohacking my own biology. This led to developing the Bulletproof Diet, at the time a radically different nutritional strategy to reach peak health, grounded in the belief that we can really take control of our own biology.

The creation of the Bulletproof Diet was not just about shedding pounds or gaining a sharper mind; it was a deep dive into how we, as humans, can reach an optimal state of being. It was about understanding how every bite of food, every decision we make, impacts our biology.

Felix has taken these principles and discovered how they can be applied to one of the world's most common inherited diseases – polycystic kidney disease – in ways that the field of medicine didn't know until now. I actually only have one kidney, so I'm very aware of how important it is to keep it healthy.

The fact that Felix is able to deduce from existing research what nobody else was able to see shows his deep understanding of biology and his scientific mind. He puts this mind to use for millions of people affected by PKD, coming up with new actionable ways to mitigate this condition, which makes this book a must-read for anyone with PKD or even other genetic conditions.

Felix's story is a vivid illustration of how the principles of biohacking can be tailored to improve even genetic conditions which some people believe to be incurable. By harnessing a state of intermittent ketosis and fasting combined with highly nutritious foods, he has uncovered a profound truth: our genetic destiny is not a script that is set in stone but a narrative that we can rewrite with the right diet, lifestyle and supplementation.

But this book is not just about his personal victory; it's a blueprint for all patients with PKD and beyond. By adapting the principles of the Bulletproof Diet to manage PKD, Felix shows the substantial role diet plays in upgrading our health. Just as I learned through my experiments and research, Felix demonstrates that the right dietary strategy can improve or, dare I say, even reverse a condition as daunting as PKD. He offers a pragmatic, science-backed approach to a complex genetic condition, underlining the power of personalized dietary strategies.

Reversing Polycystic Kidney Disease goes beyond the discouraging recommendations found at doctors' offices or on PKD websites, which are often about restrictions, medication and transplants. It introduces a proactive nutrition-focused approach to improving kidney function and even kidney size in PKD, underpinned by the same principles I developed in the Bulletproof Diet. It's a detailed exploration of the science behind PKD and ketosis and a hands-on guide to how to implement the PKDproof program, along with everything you need to know so you don't hurt yourself in the process. It cuts through the noise of confusing health recommendations and clearly highlights the fallacies in other popular approaches, making this book an invaluable resource for anyone affected by PKD looking for a solution to regain their health.

As you immerse yourself in the pages of this book, prepare for a journey that is both personal and universal. It's an exploration that challenges our understanding of what's possible, pushing the boundaries of conventional health wisdom.

Felix's story, much like my own adventures in biohacking, is an example of the incredible potential that lies within each of us to transform our health and our lives.

Dave Asprey
Founder, Bulletproof
New York Times Best-Selling Author
Pioneer of Biohacking

Preface

Hi, I'm Felix. I'm the guy who has been reversing his polycystic kidney disease (PKD) successfully since 2014. Many have followed after me since then, and now you can do so too. My glomerular filtration rate (GFR) went from its lowest point in the mid-80s to over 130 in a few years, while simultaneously my kidney volume reduced by 7% over the first three years as assessed by MRI. How did I do it? Well, hold on to your hats, because I wrote this book to teach you exactly that!

This book starts off with a deep dive into the causes of PKD and its progression, but if you want to skip all those details and just know what to do, please feel free to go straight to the 'Quick Start' guide on page 209 and the practical chapters that begin with Chapter 4, The template for the PKD program. I highly recommend you read the rest of the book though, as the more you know about your condition and your body the more motivated you will be to actually follow the guide and stick to the strategies outlined in this book.

Introduction

As you probably know, polycystic kidney disease (PKD) is one of the most common genetically inherited conditions worldwide. Up to 12 million people are affected by this mutation. There are several different types of PKD, such as ADPKD type 1 and 2, as well as ARPKD. All of these mutations lead to multiple cysts in the kidneys, but cysts can also develop in the liver, spleen, pancreas, ovaries and large bowel. Many people only get diagnosed later in life because no symptoms have been present up until that point, and many might get diagnosed by accident when getting imaging done for other reasons.

The importance of diet for PKD

For many years, as in a multitude of conditions, we have been told that there is nothing that can be done about PKD. This is what I was told when I was diagnosed at 12 years old. I got the standard advice to keep my kidneys warm, limit protein and brace for impact. Knowing that this point was far into the future, I lived most of my teenage years without thinking much about this condition, even though it always remained in the back of my mind. Asking doctors every couple of years if there had been any new developments, and then finally finding out the first medication approved for PKD only slightly slowed down the condition, I had to recognize that the medical system was probably not going to give me any answers in the near future.

In my early 20s, I began studying film directing at a German university. Throughout my studies, my stress levels steadily increased and when I was about to finish, I was in full-blown burnout. Back then, I didn't even know what to call my state of health. The only thing I knew was that getting up in the morning seemed excruciating to me and that I needed to rest.

In a very lucky chain of events, I discovered the world of podcasting and immediately proceeded to gobble up everything I could find on health and physical wellness in the hope of finding something that could remedy my situation. It didn't take long for me to find an interview with Dr Dan Kalish, introducing me to the hormonal aspects of so-called 'adrenal fatigue', which is a more scientific term for what many people call burnout.

I found an experienced practitioner well versed in treating adrenal fatigue and it took me about six months to recover. This is what got me hooked on health and from then on I proceeded to change everything in my diet and lifestyle to make it as conducive to health and longevity as I possibly could. And this is when I got the surprise information from my nephrologist, that my kidney volume had 'possibly decreased'. In the back of my mind, I had been hoping for something like this but, mind you, this was back in 2014 and nobody had discovered a link between diet and the progression of PKD at that time, nor were there any documented cases of PKD reversal.

Fast forward to today, and it turns out that, by changing my diet and lifestyle and adding targeted supplements, I have been able to reduce my kidney volume by 7% and improve my kidney function, as measured by glomerular filtration rate (GFR) from the low 80s to over 130. This has been shown in MRI scans and repeated blood tests.

Needless to say, this kind of improvement has previously been deemed impossible. If you ask your doctor, PKD only goes in one direction: downhill. Well… Maybe not anymore.

To tell the world about this, I founded a Facebook group called 'healing polycystic kidney disease naturally' and we have just (at the time of going to print) passed 5000 members. I am writing this book for anyone who suffers from this disease and is looking to improve their health and their kidney function, and possibly even reduce their cyst size or kidney volume just like I did.

My story and what is possible

Background

The standard American diet is abbreviated as 'SAD' for a reason. It's really a sad state we have come to in our society. Our foods are so far from what we evolved to eat that I can't even begin to imagine how many diseases are being caused or exacerbated by diet alone. However, some new diet paradigms have emerged over the past few years; most notably, the keto and paleo diets are gaining popularity. I myself decided to switch to a version of those back in 2014. I was suffering from severe heart arrhythmias from mold toxicity and 'burnout' (or adrenal fatigue, as explained) and was looking to make some significant changes in my life. The diet that I adopted was called the Bulletproof Diet and it's the cleverest implementation of a ketogenic diet that I have come across. It is very detailed in the foods that are in the red (avoid) and green (good to eat) zones and whatever you decide to eat, you always know where you stand.

After being on the Bulletproof Diet for a long time, I was feeling better than I had for years, in addition to the stellar results I got at my nephrologist visit. This led me to investigate why this diet and lifestyle regimen might have worked and I began to delve deep into the scientific literature. Four years later, a team at UC Santa Barbara also found this mechanism, which was then published in a 2019 study on animal models of PKD.[1]

What next?

Before we go into the 'how' of the PKDprogram or discuss any other studies in detail, let's get some basic biology and underlying science out of the way.

Throughout this book you will find three different types of evidence: my personal experience (matching that of many others), basic molecular mechanisms, and initial studies on animals as well as human studies directly investigating the effects of a ketogenic state for PKD.

To both my parents, who always believed in me.
Thank you for making me feel that anything is possible.

Chapter 1

What is PKD and why do some get it worse than others?

So, before we delve deep into how to reverse PKD, let's get some basic biology and underlying science out of the way.

The mutation

There are two main types of PKD: autosomal dominant PKD and autosomal recessive PKD.

Autosomal dominant PKD is caused by a change or mutation in either the PKD1 or PKD2 gene. This type of PKD is passed down from a parent to their child and only one copy of the changed gene is needed for the disease to develop.

Autosomal recessive PKD is caused by changes in both copies of the PKHD1 gene. This type of PKD is less common and occurs when a person inherits two changed copies of the gene, one from each parent. This book will be mostly focusing on the dominant form; however, I would encourage you to make your own experiments with the strategies in this book if you are affected by the recessive form as well.

PKD1 encodes polycystin-1 (PC-1), a large 'integral membrane protein'. This means it is permanently part of the cell membrane. Membrane proteins are part of cellular processes, including signaling, transport and maintaining the structure of the cell. In the case of the polycystin proteins, they also help cells 'stick together' as they play a role in cell adhesion.

PKD2 encodes polycystin-2 (PC-2), which is a 'transient receptor potential calcium ion channel', meaning it helps to control calcium levels inside the cell. You can think of PC-2 as a gate that opens and closes to let a specific amount of calcium ions into the cell, while PC-1 is a sensor that controls this gate and decides when to open or close it, depending on several factors, including intracellular oxygen levels. Cells need to have sufficient internal calcium levels to efficiently use oxygen for energy production, a process known as 'respiration'. However, since the PKD mutations result in less calcium making it into the cells, it impairs their ability to use oxygen and produce energy. This leads to a continuous state of low cellular energy, which over time results in the effects I will now describe.

Effects on the kidneys

Cells that have the PC-1 and PC-2 proteins in their membranes are found primarily in the kidneys but also in other parts of the body, including the liver, pancreas, blood vessels and heart.

When either of the PKD genes has a mutation that is 'expressed', meaning the genetic code is actually being used to make the proteins it encodes, it can affect how cells develop, grow and respond, as well as how accurately they can maintain their intracellular calcium levels. So over the long term, a mutation in either of the proteins can lead to a chronic calcium-deficiency state within cells, suppressing their ability to efficiently produce energy using respiration. This is the key point to understanding PKD. If cells are unable to efficiently produce energy using respiration, over the long term they revert to their ancient, prehistoric alternative mode of energy production: fermentation. For this, they can use one of two fermentable fuels: glucose or glutamine. These processes are called 'aerobic glycolysis' and 'glutaminolysis' respectively, and they are the prime characteristics of cystic cells as well as of tumors, and even cells in other diseases of uncontrolled proliferation like endometriosis, benign prostatic hyperplasia (prostate enlargement), and others. In the case of PKD, this increased intake of glucose (and, by extension, likely glutamine) seems to be part of the reason for fluid accumulation: with more fermentable fuels, by osmosis the cells also pull in more fluid, which then accumulates,[1] forming a cyst, pulling in and trapping all sorts of other substances inside with it.

Knowing that these cells are dependent on fermentation for energy also exposes their Achilles heel, which is their continuous access to fermentable fuels (glucose and glutamine). Restricting access to these fuels while keeping the rest of the body's healthy cells thriving will be a core strategy in this book.

Effects on the gut lining

Our gut lining is what separates the contents of our intestines and large bowel from our blood supply. There is a thin layer of cells deciding at all times what to absorb and what to keep in the gut for later excretion. This layer of cells is held together by so-called 'tight junctions'. Now these tight junctions can become compromised through different types of insults/traumas in our daily life; some of the worst offenders are gluten (the protein in wheat and some other grains) and other lectins. Spices such as black pepper and chili can also damage it, as well as alcohol, artificial sweeteners, trans-fats (fats damaged by over-heating) and so on.

When the tight junctions don't close properly, this is called 'leaky gut'.

Now with the PKD mutation affecting membrane proteins, the composition of the tight junctions is altered, so it stands to reason that PKD patients might be especially prone to acquiring leaky gut. Once this happens, toxins from the gut have an easy way to get into the bloodstream and finally to the kidneys where they then can cause injury, ultimately increasing cyst growth.

This means that keeping the integrity of our gut lining optimal should be one of the top priorities for any PKD patient.

Effects on blood vessels

The fact that membrane proteins are altered in PKD patients also gives patients a higher propensity for all kinds of issues related to the elasticity of our body tissues, as the mutation gives our tissues increased elasticity. This can result in cysts in the kidneys or liver, where there is ample fluid secretion, but it may also be expressed in other areas of the body, leading to the following issues, among others:

- Aneurysms: weakened blood vessels (usually arteries) that bulge and can burst, leading to serious bleeding.
- Heart valve prolapse: a condition where one or more heart valves don't close properly.
- Arterial dissection: a tear in the inner lining of an artery.
- Aortic root dilatation: a condition where the main blood vessel (aorta) from the heart becomes enlarged

There is reason to believe, that the measures proposed in this book could have a positive impact not only on cyst growth but also on these other problems, as we are addressing the pathology resulting from the mutation at its root.

Chapter 2

Basic molecular mechanisms of PKD

Why do PKD cells grow and keep growing?

It is not known how many people out there actually carry the PKD mutation without ever exhibiting actual cyst growth. However, there are some studies suggesting that PKD mutations are more common than previously suspected based on imaging data alone.[1] Lifestyle factors may in fact be the main difference between a hypothetical person carrying the PKD mutation without any symptoms and someone exhibiting classical PKD. When we are born, most of us don't express any cysts in the kidney or liver even though we carry the mutation. What's happening here?

Injury

There is something called the 'second-hit model'. This model basically dictates that if one of your chromosomes still carries a functional version of the PKD1 or PKD2 gene, initially your body might be able to silence the incorrect one, or if it expresses just 50% correctly this still might be sufficient for normal function. However, when there is injury to a specific kidney cell or liver cell later in life, it can lead to a new mutation in the healthy copy of the gene. Now the affected cell has only mutated versions of the gene left, so that is what it expresses. According to the second-hit model, only then do we actually begin to see cyst growth.[2]

Now, what does 'cell injury' actually mean? Like all cells, kidney cells can be injured by a wide variety of overt (actual physical trauma) and hidden factors, including stress, ionizing and/or non-ionizing radiation and toxic chemicals, such as the herbicide glyphosate (Roundup). They can also be injured by ROS (radical oxygen species) produced by damaged mitochondria in neighboring cystic cells, contributing to a type of domino-effect. In general, all mitochondrial and DNA-damaging toxins are of concern. To learn more about hidden sources of injury, refer to page 158.

Now, what happens as a result? What are some of the differences that we can observe between healthy kidney cells and PKD cells? An important main difference is in their metabolic function. PKD cells behave similarly to most cancer cells, fueling their growth through metabolism without oxygen.

The Warburg effect

Healthy cells make energy inside their little power plants called mitochondria. They take in energy substrates like glucose and combine them with oxygen to create energy in the form of ATP. This is a very efficient process and produces a lot of energy. This energy can then be used by the cell.

In the same process the mitochondria also produce NADH, which is an essential 'coenzyme' involved in electron transport. Think of ATP as the gasoline that keeps cells going, while NAD+ (made from NADH) is the oil of the engine, and NADH is used up oil that can be recycled. NAD+ is also the oil that greases the rapid cyst growth in PKD. Cells expressing the PKD mutation have an upregulated recycling mechanism (the enzyme lactate dehydrogenase or 'LDH'), so most of the NADH that is produced gets converted to NAD+, which makes it all the more important to keep NADH production at bay. The ratio of ATP to NADH is high in healthy aerobic metabolism ('respiration', i.e., using oxygen). In fact, slightly more than three molecules of ATP are

(a) Respiration (with oxygen)

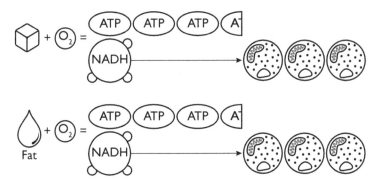

(b) Glycolysis (without oxygen) ⟶ **the Warburg effect**

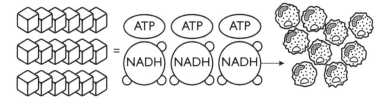

(c) Glutaminolysis (without oxygen and without glucose)

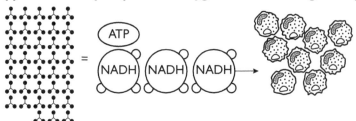

Figure 1: Glycolysis and glutaminolysis versus aerobic metabolism showing relative ATP to NADH production (NB: This is a ratio, not an absolute number)

produced for every molecule of NADH. This yields a total of 36-38 molecules of ATP and 10 molecules of NADH for every molecule of glucose, or 21.5 molecules of ATP and 6.5 molecules of NADH on average for every ketone (see Figure 1, which illustrates these proportions).

When an individual cell starts expressing the PKD mutation after the second copy of the gene mutates due to injury, or mitochondria are sufficiently harmed, the cell switches its metabolism to fermentation processes called 'aerobic glycolysis' and 'glutaminolysis', meaning it will ferment glucose (glycolysis) or glutamine (glutaminolysis) in the presence of oxygen, without actually using the oxygen. Glycolysis takes place in the body of the cell itself, without using the mitochondria. This is way less efficient than using oxygen in the process (respiration), but that is not the only problem: metabolizing one molecule of glucose only reaps a measly two molecules of ATP, but also two molecules of NADH. This means the cell is starving for energy and needs to crank up the speed of this reaction almost 20-fold to get the same amount of energy per second that it would've gotten through respiration.

This fallback process now produces a lot more NADH, which is then quickly recycled to NAD+ in mutated cells and acts as miracle-grow for cell proliferation and cyst growth. You could also say it removes the rate-limiting effect that ATP generated through respiration usually has on fueling cell growth.

Another way to think of it is that PKD cells need NADH to recycle so they can fuel their growth, but have to use up energy in the form of ATP before producing more. The more energy is produced from the substrate, the longer it takes for the cell to grow. This is called the Warburg effect and it is what happens in the growth of most cancers. Named after its discoverer, Nobel prize-winner Otto Warburg, the Warburg effect describes this metabolic shift present in most cancer cells, relying on glycolysis and glutaminolysis (instead of the more efficient oxygen-based

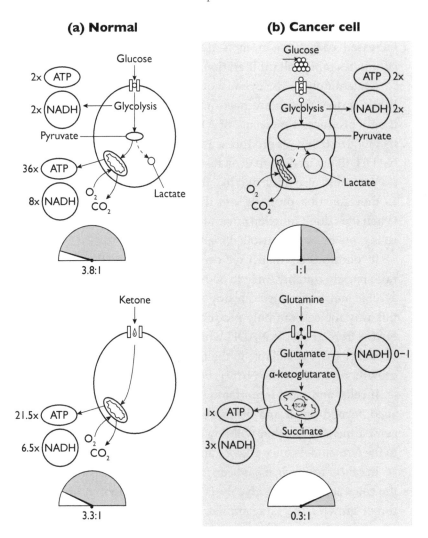

Figure 2: The Warburg effect - Comparison of cellular energy production in cells with healthy and damaged mitochondria. Healthy mitochondria metabolize glucose or ketones with oxygen into high amounts of energy in the form of ATP, while only outputting low amounts of NADH. Damaged mitochondria don't produce any energy, so the cell switches to fermentation of either glucose or glutamine, producing high amounts of NADH in the process, fueling growth.

respiration), which leads to increased NADH production and increased conversion from NADH to NAD+, which in turn stimulates rapid cell proliferation.

Glutaminolysis is even worse than aerobic glycolysis. While it does take place even inside damaged mitochondria, it only produces 1 molecule of ATP per molecule of glutamine metabolized, but it produces a whopping 3-4 molecules of NADH, likely leading to even faster cell growth.

You could also think of it like this: our mitochondria, as long as they function properly, are the controllers of cell growth. When they don't function anymore, the brakes are disabled and cells grow in an uncontrolled manner.

It follows then, that if we can increase the ATP to NADH ratio back to roughly three to one by switching the cells back to aerobic metabolism, we can stop rapid growth of PKD cells, as this way the cell can only produce a much smaller amount of NAD+ from available NADH while using up the large amount of energy that is available in the form of ATP – in other words, growth, proportional to NAD+, becomes normal again.

If cells, and most importantly their mitochondria, are damaged beyond repair and therefore are unable to switch back to aerobic metabolism, they will slowly die off as long as their access to the fermentable fuels glucose and glutamine is restricted.

In cancer research, it has been found that chemically blocking the cell's ability to use glycolysis is a valuable tool in limiting tumor growth. The same applies to PKD cells. If we can block any of the steps needed to perform glycolysis while providing everything needed for aerobic metabolism, the cell will have no other option than to revert to healthy aerobic metabolism or die. Now, while cancer researchers are using different chemicals to reach this state and are having some success with this approach, we are of course interested in sustainable natural methods to do so and are looking for approaches with the lowest risk but the highest possible reward.

Blocking glucose uptake

This is where ketones come into play. Ketones are your body's alternative fuel source to glucose. I'm sure you've heard of blood glucose; ketones are the alternative. Glucose comes from carbohydrates like sugar and starch or from glycogen stores, mostly in the muscles and liver. In contrast, ketones are produced from stored body fat or dietary fats, at least if your body is trained to do it. This is called ketosis.

So how do we use ketones to our advantage in PKD? They simply cannot be metabolized without oxygen (anaerobically), so whenever a PKD cell metabolizes ketones instead of glucose, it switches back to healthy aerobic metabolism or dies.

Aerobic metabolism is great for energy, but not great for uncontrolled cell proliferation that leads to cyst growth. In other words, ketones block the Warburg effect by switching the cell's energy metabolism to using oxygen, producing more than three molecules of ATP for every molecule of NADH, and thereby exhibiting a sort of time-release effect for the cell's production and usage of NAD+, which is needed for growth.

Some researchers have seen good results from blocking glucose uptake altogether, which can force PKD cells into suicide. While researchers are using patentable drugs like 2DG to achieve this, Mother Nature has prepared a similar molecule with very few side effects: ascorbic acid, also known as vitamin C. Vitamin C has a structure strikingly similar to glucose and can be taken up by our cells. Some research has shown that high-dose vitamin C actually interferes with the Warburg effect by blocking the flow of energy.

Now, it is true that vitamin C is metabolized to oxalic acid, which in turn can increase the risk of kidney stones. The scientific literature is quite divided on this, but it makes sense to take care of one's own urine pH balance to prevent stone formation altogether. We will go into this in further detail later in the book (page 152). It should be noted that humans are among the only mammals, except for guinea pigs, certain primates and bats, that do not produce their own vitamin C from glucose.

For reference, a healthy ape the same size as a human will produce somewhere around 2000 to 4000 mg of vitamin C on a normal day, whereas goats, being among the highest producers of vitamin C, can produce up to 100,000 mg per day when they are sick. Of course, it would make sense to distribute any kind of supplementation throughout the day to mimic natural production; just keep in mind that all antioxidants like vitamin C break a fast and therefore should only be taken in the 'eating window' of your daily schedule (often called the 'feeding window' in research). I describe this schedule and how to balance eating with fasting to reverse PKD on page 90.

Promoting autophagy and suppressing mTOR

It turns out that there are multiple molecular mechanisms at work in producing the cysts that manifest in PKD. One of the most important ones is 'mTOR', short for 'mammalian target of rapamycin' (a common immunosuppressive drug with surprising health benefits), a signal to the body to build new tissues, be it for repair, growing cysts or building muscle. mTOR is needed for cyst growth to take place, much like NAD+, but it is also needed to repair damaged tissues and prevent muscle loss. Consequently, the only rational approach seems to be to activate it sometimes and inhibit it at other times. That is the effect of intermittent fasting, which I describe in detail later. Whenever you fast for somewhere between 12 and 18 hours, mTOR begins to be inhibited, and cysts slow or stop their growth, depending on how much mTOR inhibition is going on. Concurrently, the opposite mechanism is then activated, which is called autophagy.[3, 4]

The term 'autophagy' has its origin in Greek and means 'eating oneself'. Whenever you inhibit mTOR and thereby activate autophagy, your body scours all the tissues for damaged proteins and damaged mitochondria – the power-plants of your cells as mentioned above. This is fortunate because PKD tissues are damaged, both from a protein and a mitochondrial perspective. This means, that whenever autophagy is active, your body will gobble up PKD-affected cells. Whenever that happens, the damaged cells are gobbled up and dissolved into their individual amino acids, which can then be a source for building new and healthy tissues. Sounds good, right?

So why don't we do this all the time? Why don't we fast all the time? Well, simply put, fasting indefinitely is also called starving to death. So that obviously will not work. However, we can employ the technique of intermittent fasting and get the benefits of autophagy for a couple of hours every day, while using mTOR to rebuild our tissues later.

Over a long period, this dance can significantly improve your kidney function and even volume, as it has mine and that of many others. However, there are of course many factors that increase cyst growth and, if you don't take care of these, you might not be able to tip the scales in your favor. Our goal has to be to remove as many cyst-promoting factors as we can while simultaneously getting enough autophagy to remove more cystic tissue than we are building.

Slowing cyst growth with ketones

So now that we know what gets our kidneys to shrink, what do we have to remove from our lives to slow cyst growth while we are in our eating window?

The science will probably never be complete in this area since human studies on lifestyle factors are few and far between and very difficult to conduct. The most prudent approach to the matter is therefore to remove as many things as possible that negatively impact human health and performance in general, while maximizing the autophagy we are getting in our fasting window.

One of the ways to slow the metabolism and thereby the growth of these damaged PKD cells is to become 'fat adapted' and run most of our body's metabolism on ketones, the alternative fuel to glucose mentioned above.

Ketones are an essential part of fueling the human body. We actually come into this world in a state of ketosis, but in our current society we eat large amounts of carbohydrates daily, which can lead to high blood glucose and the loss of the ability to metabolize ketones in the long term. We call this a state of metabolic inflexibility.

When you start on a ketogenic diet there is an adaptation window of a few weeks to up to three months that you need for your body to fully adapt and develop the ability to metabolize ketones as fuel. Once you have reached this stage called 'fat adaptation' you will be able to go without food for prolonged periods of time and you will feel less of a need to eat frequently. Instead, you will feel relaxed around food and be able to decide if you are going to eat or not. It will make it far easier to stick to the intermittent fasting regimen that I am recommending.

Bulletproof coffee

To make it even easier, and even add some additional benefits to the diet, in the mornings, instead of your traditional breakfast you will have a delicious cup of 'bulletproof coffee'. That is, a cup of coffee made from mold-free beans that have been lab tested (you don't want any mold toxins from your coffee burdening your kidneys every day) combined with a tablespoon or more of grass-fed butter and a tablespoon or more of MCT oil, preferably from a glass bottle and with at least 60% C8 content. ('MCT' stands for 'medium-chain triglycerides', a type of fat found in coconut and palm oil. Check out the manufacturer's description to make sure.) Some preliminary data suggest a dose of around 18 grams of C8 yields the highest increase in blood ketones, which is around 0.5 mmol/l.[5]

I have been drinking bulletproof coffee on the majority of my mornings since I started on this diet and, in my research, I then discovered many distinct mechanisms that explain why exactly this drink might be so powerful. More on those later in the section on why bulletproof coffee works (see page 55).

Confirmation: The first study

Now, after I had already started seeing positive results from people all over the world, plus receiving a whole lot of skepticism from medical and patient advocate groups, finally the first study investigating the glucose-dependent mechanisms of PKD was published. This research by J. A. Torres and colleagues[6] was the first to investigate the effects of ketosis on the progression of PKD, albeit in an animal model – in other words, not in humans in a real-life situation. It finally confirmed that the mechanisms I've described really are at play and it demonstrated that ketosis, induced through either a ketogenic diet or intermittent or acute fasting, can actually inhibit cyst growth in PKD animal models. The study confirmed that ketosis likely works by exploiting the metabolic inflexibility of cystic cells, also called the Warburg effect, as described above. The researchers agreed that this inflexibility led to the observed reduction in cyst volume and progression. They continued by adding that the ketogenic state inhibits mTOR signaling, essential for cell proliferation and thereby cyst growth in affected kidneys.

One of the most important findings of the study was that ketosis was able to reduce cyst growth and improve kidney function even in rats in an advanced stage of PKD. This suggests that ketosis might be a viable treatment option for people at all stages of PKD.

So, knowing all this, let's continue to elaborate on mechanisms we can influence in PKD and how to do it.

Reducing glutamine levels

Now that we've discussed the uptake and metabolism of glucose as the primary fuel for cyst growth, let's turn again to this slightly more recent advance in the area of cancer metabolism that applies to PKD, adding a critical part to this puzzle. While restricting glucose is the most important part of reversing PKD as it creates the environment for cyst growth to slow down or even go into reverse, as you already know by now, there is another fuel that cysts can use to grow: glutamine.

Glutamine is an amino acid which is integral to our body's function. While most of our healthy cells have evolved to do just fine without glucose whenever ketones are present, glutamine is so essential that our bodies make sure levels in the blood are mostly stable, independent of dietary factors. Glutamine is needed for all sorts of bodily functions, most importantly the immune system. When glutamine is low, immune cells are paralyzed and the risk of infection runs high. Cancer cells and even PKD cells use this to their advantage by fermenting glutamine to, among other things, make energy, very similar to fermenting glucose in aerobic glycolysis.

Professor Thomas N. Seyfried discovered this missing link in cancer therapy and subsequently published the paper, 'Press-pulse: a novel therapeutic strategy for the metabolic management of cancer'.[7] In this paper, he outlines the need for combining glucose-lowering diets like the Bulletproof Diet, which he calls a 'press' on the cancer, with strategic 'pulses', meaning short bursts of extreme stress on the cells in the body, which will then selectively target and affect the weakest cells. The cancer cells in Seyfried's case being the only ones unable to use ketones for their energy needs, will then be the first to die, as their secondary fuel, glutamine, is being restricted by the 'pulse' intervention. Giving cells the 'pulse' on its own, without the 'press' environment will yield far inferior results. The combination of both is key, as the cells can otherwise get their energy from the fuel that is not restricted.

It's important to understand, that, contrary to glucose, healthy cells will always need glutamine. Consequently, constant, extreme lowering of glutamine levels is impossible. As previously mentioned, proper levels are needed for many functions in the body, such as the synthesis of proteins, the production of antioxidants like glutathione, and the support of the immune system's ability to fight infections. Glutamine also plays a crucial role in maintaining the integrity of the intestinal lining, preventing harmful bacteria and toxins from leaking into the bloodstream — which is another important point we will return to later (see page 146).

All of this research in cancer, it turns out, is highly relevant for PKD. A 2018 paper found there are similar changes to glutamine metabolism in PKD cells.[8] This makes sense as their growth and energy production patterns, as well as mitochondrial changes, are strikingly similar to those of cancer, as we discussed already.

What then is the 'pulse' intervention? Since no dietary intervention can lower glutamine levels much over the long term, this is one area where specific drugs and supplements are the only option. Glutamine levels can be lowered by inhibiting several different enzymes that are involved in its metabolism. The strongest drug is DON (6-diazo-5-oxo-L-norleucine), a glutamine analog (meaning its structure resembles that of glutamine). Because of its structure, it acts on a multitude of pathways involved in glutamine metabolism, efficiently inhibiting glutamine uptake. Sadly, at the moment DON is mostly used by researchers and only a very few cancer patients, which makes it quite expensive. It's also dangerous to dose DON without knowing exactly what to do, as, among other things, the immune system becomes acutely paralyzed.

Since the options for lowering glutamine blood levels are quite limited, we will focus on limiting glucose, increasing ketones and targeting additional mechanisms through diet and supplements for most of this book. However, some strategies and drugs to limit glutamine will be discussed later in the chapter on supplements and medications (page 152).

Exercising to optimize intermittent fasting

While intermittent fasting is a cornerstone of our approach to reduce cyst growth, a 2018 study by Dethlefsen and colleagues went into further detail in assessing how effective it really is, and the key take-away from that study was that the effectiveness of intermittent fasting highly depends on your fitness.[3] Let me explain. When you fast, your body quickly gets to a state of nutrient deficiency, which is why it needs to tap into its stores. This goes for all nutrients. For example, your body needs to consume at least enough calories to keep your basic functions going, which is why you will lose weight when fasting. Optimally, you would lose body fat and convert it into energy.

Now, the cyst walls in PKD aren't made of fat, as you probably know; they're made of protein. So naturally when we want to reduce cysts, we need to be in a protein-deficient state. When our bodies are not actively building up tissues, there is not a high requirement for protein so this protein-deficiency state can slowly build up within an intermittent fasting window. That 2018 study showed that autophagy slowly starts increasing around the 36-hour mark in 'untrained' individuals, meaning those not in the top 25% of their age group for fitness.[3]

Now, this leads us to a huge realization: the effectiveness of an intermittent fast is highly dependent on how much we exercise. People who performed in the top 25% of their age group in terms of fitness (which is what the researchers called

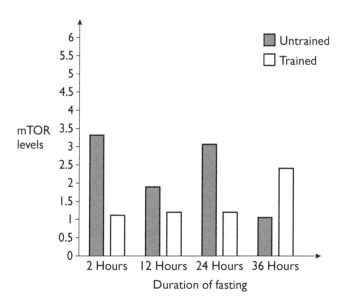

Figure 3: Comparison of the degree of mTOR inhibition between people who exercise regularly and those who do not: The chart shows mTOR levels in study participants after different durations of fasting. Lower is better, meaning more autophagy, e.g. more dissolution of damaged proteins. Untrained individuals took 36 hours of fasting to reach levels of 1.0, while trained individuals took just two hours.

'trained') started seeing the benefits of autophagy during the fast very quickly, starting even as soon as the two-hour mark. It took people who did not exercise enough to be considered in the top 25% a whopping 36 hours to reach the same level of mTOR inhibition that the trained subjects got after two hours of fasting. This makes intuitive sense because individuals who train regularly need lots of protein to repair and build muscle, while individuals who do not are just in maintenance mode, making their protein demands lower. The time it takes for actual protein deficiency to occur is therefore a lot higher.

The researchers defined 'trained' people as being the top 25% (75th percentile) of their age group in terms of fitness as measured by their maximum oxygen uptake during training. This value is also called **VO$_2$ max**. To get an accurate reading of your VO$_2$ max, some fitness centers and clinics offer a test that is usually done on a stationary bike with an oxygen mask that measures how much oxygen you're actually taking up. A test like this can be pretty costly so you can employ an alternative option. If you're sedentary, you can just use the simple formula below: put in your age and resting heart rate (HRrest). Measure this with a sleep tracker, smart watch or manually after sitting down for a couple of minutes.

$$VO_2 \text{ max} = 15 \times (220\text{-age/HRrest})$$

So, to spell it out, subtract your age from 220, divide that by your resting heart rate and multiply the result by 15.

If you want a more accurate way to test using a stationary treadmill or a digital map, you can use the 'Cooper 1.5 Mile Run Test'. It will give you a more accurate measurement without breaking the bank: find out how long it takes you to run 1.5 miles as fast as possible (2.4 km). Either use a treadmill or use a digital map to measure out a track for you to run. Then you can calculate your VO$_2$ max as follows:

$$VO_2 \text{ max} = (483/\text{time}) + 3.5^4$$

There are also some smart watches on the market that estimate your VO$_2$ max. An honorable mention goes to the Garmin models and the Apple Watch, as these come from the only manufacturers that regularly offer an option to turn off Bluetooth so you are not stressing your body with EMFs during your run. To save money, you can get an older used model that just does heart rate and calculate the results yourself.

Table 1: Estimated threshold for autophagy to begin depending on age extrapolated from marathon times of elite runners

Age	20	25	30	35	40	45	50	55	60	65	70	75	80	85	90
VO_2 max threshold male	55	55	55	55	53	51	48	46	43	41	38	35	31	26	20
VO_2 max threshold female	45	45	45	45	44	42	39	36	33	31	28	25	21	17	11

Source: VO_2 max thresholds for optimal autophagy are extrapolated based on declining elite runner marathon speeds over age, starting from the known point of 55/ml/min at 25-30 years.[9]

Table 1 represents an estimate of where the threshold for autophagy for each age group may lie. We only know the definite value in the 25-30 age group; all other values are based on the assumption that the threshold follows the same curve that VO_2 max in athletes follows over time. Now if you don't find yourself above the threshold of your gender and age group, most people can definitely get there with enough training. One HIRT heavy-weight-training session per week as outlined later in this book (page 135), one to two HIRT cardio training sessions and daily brisk walks or an extended hike on the weekends can go a long way towards reaching your threshold VO_2 max. Of course this is likely a sliding scale, so every improvement in the right direction is worthwhile. You will be able to harness the benefits of intermittent fasting in a much more pronounced way, because you will be using up protein more quickly to build muscle. This will force your body into autophagy quickly when you're fasting, dissolving injured kidney tissues multiple times faster than it would otherwise. With the right exercise regimen, you can expect improvements in VO_2 max after two to 12 months, depending on where you're starting from.[10] You can find details on how to train later in this book (page 135).

What if I don't exercise?

Of course it's up to you if you exercise or not and how much. The study mentioned above makes it extremely clear that exercise with fasting is multiple times more powerful than fasting alone. To say it more clearly: to get the benefits of a daily 16-hour intermittent fast in a trained person, an untrained person would have to fast for 52 hours. The difference is that monumental. So if you are able, there's really no excuse not to increase your VO_2 max starting today.

If you are overweight, or for some other reason cannot immediately begin raising your cardiovascular fitness this way, it would be very sensible to include a three-day protein fast once a month or a two-day protein fast twice a month to get considerable levels of autophagy going regularly. This is not to say that intermittent fasting is not an essential part of the diet even for untrained individuals, as the alternative would be to eat for a longer period of time, which would increase mTOR and therefore cyst growth during the day for longer periods of time than necessary with normal food consumption.

Molecular triggers

The initial PKD mutation leads to many different imbalances and to changes in a multitude of pathways in the body. Some of them can be positively impacted by over-the-counter supplements and dietary strategies. I call them molecular triggers. Some of the most prominent and easy to influence ones include:

- Autophagy
- mTOR
- AMPK
- NAD+
- SIRT1
- HDACs

- Intracellular calcium (Ca^{2+})
- p53
- TNF-alpha

Some of these mechanisms interact with and modify each other – for example, inhibition of mTOR directly leads to autophagy, which tends to clean up mutated cells in PKD kidneys. So, autophagy acts as a cellular clean-up crew, helping to eliminate unnecessary components and limit cell growth, and mTOR is like a fuel pump for cell growth, including necessary growth such as muscle cells, as well as growth of mutated PKD cells. Most people nowadays live in a constant state of mTOR activation and therefore never experience autophagy. Stopping food intake for somewhere around 12-18 hours has been shown to increase autophagy,[11, 12] making this mechanism a great target for diet and supplements to positively influence PKD.

AMPK is an enzyme that is involved in energy regulation of the cell. Activating AMPK inhibits mTOR, which then activates autophagy. You can think of it as a see-saw effect.

SIRT1 is a gene-regulating enzyme, which exists in a tight relationship with AMPK. SIRT1 is also an intermediate for NAD+ to exhibit its cyst growth-promoting effect. Unsurprisingly, studies have shown that inhibition of SIRT1 led to inhibition of cyst growth in mice.[13] However, efforts to try and inhibit SIRT1 directly in the whole body to limit cyst growth would adversely impact longevity and long-term health, so this is not a strategy we will explore further. There are supplements on the market that claim to boost SIRT1 for longevity effects, like resveratrol, but there has been some controversy around these claims.[14]

HDACs (histone-deacetylases) are a class of enzymes that regulate gene expression, including the genes implicated in PKD. They also influence the calcium signal triggered by fluid flow in kidney epithelial cells. Cystic epithelial cells tend to show increased levels of HDAC6 expression[15] and researchers have discovered that inhibiting multiple HDACs can reduce the formation of cysts[16] and slow down the decline of kidney function in a mouse study modeling human PKD.

Optimizing your epigenetics

Epigenetics is the science of how your lifestyle and external as well as internal environment influence the expression of your genes. Since PKD is a genetic disease, this field should be of particular interest to us. You see, it's not as much about the genes we are born with as we are led to believe. It is more about the genes that we currently express. And we do have some wriggle room here.

There is research that is showing the inhibition of certain HDACs to be beneficial. Now, we can't hit all HDACs that were targeted in studies with food and supplements for now, but at least some of them we can.

There are several classes of HDAC. Most notably, class I HDAC inhibition has shown promising results in PKD. One potent inhibitor of class I HDAC is butyric acid, also known as butyrate, which is a type of ketone, and the most prominent ketone, beta-hydroxybutyrate (BHB) can do it, too. Besides upregulating your blood ketones, butyrate is also produced by gut bacteria when they metabolize vegetables and even apple cider vinegar.

Why didn't my doctor tell me this?

After hearing about all the different mechanisms and options to start addressing PKD from different angles, you might be wondering why you haven't heard about any of these from your family doctor or nephrologist. The answer is simple: they don't know. Why don't they know? In our current medical system, doctors get the bulk of their education upfront, in medical schools that are mostly funded by the pharmaceutical industry where the emphasis is on pharmaceutical treatments. Therefore, nutritional interventions and even most supplements are barely talked about, if not actually deemed dangerous. Continuing education in these areas exists, but isn't mandatory. In this environment, there is little incentive to learn more about nutritional approaches, especially since doctors might even get sued if they don't offer the official standard of care. Also, it is generally not the doctor's role to try out new approaches, since they usually rely on information that has filtered through to them from published research; again, much of this is funded by the pharmaceutical industry so is inevitably biased towards treatment with drugs.

The pharmaceutical industry on the other hand has little interest in developing methods to heal your condition for good. It is more incentivized to make your condition tolerable, so that you will come back for more. Some readers will have come to this realization a long time ago, while others might still be oblivious to this fact.

Western pharmaceutical- and surgery-based medicine is usually highly effective for addressing infections and acute trauma. That's where we are seeing great results. Most doctors are usually not qualified to give nutritional advice or equipped to address the causes of chronic conditions.

But even if your doctor is one of the few that is actually open to alternative strategies, how would they know about this new approach? There have been very few studies investigating the effect of the ketogenic diet on PKD. In fact, when I started writing about this, there were zero studies. Some evidence already existed in the scientific literature, but it needed to be put together by somebody who saw the parallels between other conditions – like cancer and PKD – and the evidence for different treatment methods. Generally, your doctor is not going to have time to spend days or weeks reading studies about your condition to find a new approach. That is what patients have to do.

And even now that we are seeing results in PKD patients who are actually reducing their kidney volume and increasing kidney function, these results are often times brushed aside as being anecdotal. Mind you, anecdotal evidence is still evidence, but it's going to take a long time before there are large double-blind placebo-controlled studies on ketosis in PKD, much less on a ketogenic diet, which is pretty hard to design a placebo for, considering you know what you're putting in your mouth when you're eating.

So, anecdotal evidence and animal models are all we have for now and it might stay that way for some time. You can ask your doctor what they think you should do. Wait on the sidelines until your function declines to the point of needing dialysis? Or go ahead and try what's been working for other patients anecdotally and find out for yourself? You're going to have to eat food anyway, so it might as well be the right food. Your doctor's answer will show you what their priorities are.

Understanding balance

In our bodies, there is a delicate balance between growth and breakdown, between building new tissues and getting rid of old and damaged ones, keeping everything just right. Well, at least there should be. This balance, however, has long been lost to our unnatural relationship with food.

Let's be real. Most of society is eating for the majority of the day. They get up, they have breakfast, then there is a snack, lunch, another snack, dinner, some more snacks, and finally, they go to bed for too little sleep just to get up and eat again. Most people only stop eating when they sleep. And I was the same.

However, our bodies did not evolve to live this way. We used to have periods of scarcity, even starvation. And evolution came up with a clever way to make use of these periods. Whenever there was little food, our bodies switched into autophagy, as mentioned above. Little molecules called lysosomes traveled around the bloodstream and gobbled up proteins that they could then reuse to build new tissues. Which proteins did they gobble up? They were looking for damaged proteins that were no longer working, which our body neatly tags whenever they are discovered. Even in healthy people, up to 30% of proteins are misfolded right from the time they are produced, so there is a lot of damage to be repaired.

Because we don't experience these times of starvation anymore, these damaged proteins now instead accumulate over years and decades and gum up our whole system; they lead to warts, skin blemishes, abscesses, tumors and much more. A cyst inside a PKD kidney contains a lot of that damaged protein. So is it being dissolved by the lysosomes? It does not seem that way considering the unrelenting growth seen in most PKD patients. So what's up with the lysosomes? After all, that's their job, right?

We are simply eating too frequently. A period of scarcity is recognized by our body whenever we stop eating for 15 hours or longer. So it's not about how much we eat, but rather when we eat.

The sweet spot for intermittent fasting seems to be somewhere between 15 and 18 hours of fasting per day on most days, especially when you are metabolically fit. Multiple days of protein fasting might be required for people who don't exercise regularly, as we've seen (page 21). When we trigger autophagy like that, we restore this delicate balance between growth and breakdown. And this is where we begin to tip the scales a little further in our favor so that ultimately we may be able to break down a little more cystic tissue during our fast than we are building up during the day.

That's the goal. If you can tip these scales in your favor, if you are able to break down more cystic tissue than you build up during any 24-hour period, you win.

This is the definition of reversing PKD.

Summary

So it's a simple formula: break down more cystic tissue while fasting than you are building up in the eating window. Remember, you will probably always be building up cystic tissues while you are eating; that's the nature of the genetic defect as far as we know it for now.

Your blood glucose level will not go below a certain level as it is tightly regulated by your body, but glucose can always be utilized to promote growth of cystic tissues. The higher your ketone levels, the lower your blood glucose can go as it is not needed by the body. The more PKD cells can metabolize ketones, the more will either revert back to a healthy state or commit suicide. Additionally, the more you trigger autophagy, the more damaged cells you will remove.

It's a delicate balance and you just have to tip it in your favor very slightly. Then you might see a slow and steady reduction in kidney volume and an increase in function over time. Everybody's different and everybody might need to do a different amount of work to tip the scales in their favor. For some people it might be very easy and they might already see results with only the ketogenic diet or intermittent fasting. Other people might have to go to greater lengths to achieve higher levels of ketones during the day. They might have to get fit, fast for longer periods to inhibit mTOR and trigger some other mechanisms overnight using strategic supplementation. The mechanisms are all laid out in this book so you can find the approach that works best for you.

Chapter 3

Looking deeper: The X factor

A mysterious substance in cyst fluid

So we have looked at injury of kidney cells earlier in this book (page 5) and we have concluded that injuring a kidney cell in a PKD patient increases the chances of this cell becoming cystic as it switches to fermentation. The next question would be: is this always the case? Or is there an instance where injuring cells over and over does not lead to cyst growth and instead the cells retain the ability to heal and revert back to their healthy state? Yes, such cases have been described in several studies and they are highly intriguing. The question then becomes, what differentiates a cell that reacts to injury with uncontrolled growth from a cell that does not?

To elucidate this, I will take you down the path of some exciting research. As long ago as 1970, Darmady and colleagues had hypothesized that the expression of cysts in PKD might be connected to a specific toxin since the changes in renal structure were found at points where toxins were 'maximally concentrated'.[1] This was followed in 1995 by experiments using extracted cyst fluid from PKD patients, applied to healthy non-PKD tissue. The researchers found that this fluid stimulated 'fluid secretion, cyclic adenosine monophosphate accumulation, and cell proliferation', which are hallmarks of

PKD, even though there was no mutation present. The toxins themselves were enough to exhibit the same effect.[2]

In the same year, a group of researchers led by JJ Grantham tried to dig deeper and used mass spectrometry to narrow the constituents of the cyst fluid down to a single substance that actually was responsible for triggering cyst growth. While they were able to concentrate the fluid to a point where its secretory activity was 48-fold above that of the original substance, meaning its ability to produce fluid that could fill a cyst was 48 times higher, they could not narrow it down to a single substance and described it as a fraction of lipids enriched in monoglycerides.[3]

Nine years before that, Avner had led a study in which he showed that complete regression of cystic changes was possible, after only 120 hours, when he removed the cell culture from its environment, thereby removing all of the present toxins as well.[4]

Endotoxin

Even though the mass spectrometry study didn't yield conclusive results and bears repeating now that our technology has evolved further, we might still be able to look at other analyses of cyst fluid from PKD kidneys to shed more light on the issue.

Miller-Hjelle and colleagues in 1997 found the substance lipopolysaccharide (LPS), also known as 'endotoxin', or its remnants in all samples of cyst fluid retrieved from human PKD kidneys. LPS, or endotoxin, is part of the outer shell of gram-negative bacteria, which shed it either chronically while they're alive or in a single large bolus upon cell death.[5]

To understand cyst growth better, we'll take a look at what researchers usually do to create cystic tissue to study. The injury that researchers need to start cyst growth is sometimes triggered by using a chemical such as NDGA (nordihydroguaiaretic acid, a kidney-toxic chemical compound). In 1987, Gardner and colleagues found that to provoke cyst growth with NDGA, they had to add endotoxin.[6] Without endotoxin, NDGA injured the kidney cells, but no cyst growth was observed.

Another breadcrumb was added to this mystery in 1990, when Miller and colleagues stated that 73% of PKD patients tested positive for endotoxiuria, meaning endotoxin excretion in urine, which 'raise[d] the possibility that endotoxin is available intrarenally to promote cystogenesis' – meaning, endotoxin is present inside the kidneys to stimulate the development of cysts.[7]

It's starting to look like there is a connection between cysts and endotoxin. Is this a PKD thing? Or is this a general cyst thing? What about other cystic diseases? Could this be the X-factor that is necessary for cyst growth and PKD progression? As it happens, both polycystic ovary syndrome (PCOS, where the cysts actually are fluid-filled follicles) and even cystic acne have been hypothesized to be connected with the presence of endotoxin.

Now, to repeat what I said above, endotoxin comes from gram-negative bacteria. But these bacteria shouldn't even be inside our kidneys or ovaries or skin in meaningful amounts, should they? Where are they coming from?

There was a paper on PCOS in 2012 by Tremellen and Pearce that hypothesized 'disturbances in bowel bacterial flora ("Dysbiosis of Gut Microbiota") brought about by a poor diet creates an increase in gut mucosal permeability, with a resultant increase in the passage of lipopolysaccharide (LPS/ endotoxin) from gram-negative colonic bacteria into the systemic circulation. [...] Thus, the Dysbiosis of Gut Microbiota (DOGMA) theory of PCOS can account for [...] the development of multiple small ovarian cysts.'[8]

So, in PCOS it might be that a poor diet gives you leaky gut and, in turn, endotoxin can permeate through the gut wall into the bloodstream and finally end up in the ovaries. Of course, this mechanism might easily translate to PKD. It might even be more likely; kidneys are our main filtration system after all.

Even worse, as we now know, the PKD mutation makes our tight junctions in the gut, which are responsible for holding in what needs to stay in and letting out what needs to get out, more permeable. The mutation gives it more elasticity, which means there is a higher amount of anything going through from the get-go.

Now, what does endotoxin bind to in our bloodstream? How do we usually mitigate this issue?

One of the molecules that endotoxin binds to in our bodies is an enzyme called argininosuccinate synthase (AS). This is one of our endotoxin shields. It's an enzyme that we need for proper excretion of excess nitrogen from protein intake, as well as for synthesizing adequate levels of the amino acids argininosuccinate and, indirectly, arginine. As it turns out, PKD patients have extremely reduced levels of this enzyme. In one rat PKD model study,[9] at 21 days old the rats already had their AS levels reduced by a staggering 90%. That's about six years old in human years. So adding insult to injury (pun intended), PKD patients don't just seem to have increased endotoxin; they also have very low levels of this enzyme needed to inactivate it, maybe because it's being used up so quickly?

So, the hypothesis would be:
- bacteria produce endotoxin, which then
- permeates through the bloodstream, where it
- can't be inactivated because of low levels of AS and
- ends up in the kidneys, causing cysts,
- triggered or potentiated by additional injury?

Maybe at least part of this has already been studied somewhere?

Luckily, there is a mouse model of germ-free mice. These

mice have been bred to have a sterile intestinal tract (poor mice) and therefore no gut flora. When in 1986 Gardner and colleagues used germ-free CFWwd mice, which are used to model human PKD, and fed them a microbe-free diet, virtually none of them developed cystic kidney disease. Since they do not possess any gut microbes, there's no source of endotoxin in these mice. Once removed from their sterile environment and given the chance to seed a gut microbial population, they began to develop cysts.[10]

Huh. This is telling us something.

While this hypothesis might be new in PKD, a very similar hypothesis has actually been well established since 2010 for liver cirrhosis. James P Nolan, in 'The role of intestinal endotoxin in liver injury' wrote: 'The overarching concept is the universality of the role of enteric endotoxin in liver injury from toxic agents. […] eliminating or reducing the enteric endotoxin pool protects the liver from injury by all such agents.'[11]

Now, why might the body react to endotoxin this way? Obviously, growing cysts in response to endotoxin is not a specific property of the PKD mutation. We discussed earlier how we have found research that shows cyst fluid can trigger cysts in non-mutated tissue.[2] There is even research that shows other kinds of cyst can be triggered by endotoxin.[12] So why does the body decide to make cysts when it comes into contact with endotoxin at injured cell sites? Is it possible that this is an ingenious form of 'the solution to pollution is dilution'? Is it possible that a cyst is a way to mitigate damage when the ability to detox endotoxin is impaired?

If that were the case, any future medication that would block cyst formation without taking care of the functional defects in the kidney cells could potentially lead to unwanted effects of toxicity or even sepsis.

The ketone connection

We have looked at the capacity of ketones to modulate PKD cyst growth already, but this might not get to the root of the issue just yet. Nolan in 2010[11] already recognized that medium-chain triglycerides, which are metabolized to ketones in the liver, could be used to reverse inflammatory and fibrotic changes in liver cirrhosis caused by endotoxin. In 2019 a study by Neudorf and colleagues showed that ketones increased the markers of NLRP3 inflammasome activation in response to endotoxin, thereby increasing the detoxification of stored endotoxin and, in turn, contributing to the drainage of cyst fluid.[13]

This would fit together with ketones' properties to be able to revert cells back to their healthy state, making them better able to process toxins.

Better therapies

Short of being able to correct the actual PKD mutation throughout the body, the next best thing seems to be finding a way to stop endotoxin from making its way to the kidneys and liver in the first place. There are several different options for achieving this.

One could try to:

1. stop the production of endotoxin in the gut or anywhere else in the body where gram-negative bacteria have colonized,
2. tighten the tight junctions in the gut lining to prevent any endotoxin from leaking into the bloodstream,
3. bind up as much endotoxin as possible with adsorbents in the bloodstream or
4. improve the body's ability to detox it when it reaches the kidney or liver tissues.

Using ketones as fuel only hits the fourth of those different approaches. It's definitely a great strategy, but what about the rest? Can we find simple, accessible, low-risk approaches to all of these points? Can we minimize the amount of endotoxin that ends up in the kidneys in the first place, to increase the effectiveness of ketosis even more?

I think we probably can. Let's take a look at what we'll be discussing next:

1. Probiotics, prebiotics, VIOME diet fine-tuning to lower endotoxin-producing bacteria's activity (see Chapter 11)
2. Glutamine and collagen supplementation (see Chapter 11), avoiding toxins through the Bulletproof Diet to tighten the tight junctions (see Chapter 4)
3. Supplementing chitosan, charcoal, cholestyramine, MCP, quercetin and fisetin, as well as up-regulating AS with citrulline to bind up endotoxin (see Chapter 11)
4. Ketones, MCT oil, milk thistle to upregulate our detox ability (see Chapter 11).

We will address each of these in more detail in the coming chapters.

Chapter 4

The template for the PKDproof program

The diet at the core of the PKDproof program is called the Bulletproof Diet (a nod to its inspiration reflected in its name). Developed by biohacker Dave Asprey, it is a cyclical version of the ketogenic diet, meaning it is interrupted by about one to three 'carbohydrate re-feed' days per week, while avoiding the most prominent antinutrients. Reaching a state of ketosis through diet, also called 'nutritional ketosis', is the magic sauce that enables our bodies to fat-adapt and produce ketones, which in turn limits kidney cyst growth by limiting access to glucose, thereby blocking glycolysis. We make it even more effective by including an intermittent fasting regimen that pushes our bodies towards autophagy most days of the week. However, both of these strategies need to be interrupted every now and then, so that we don't suffer any negative consequences, like low thyroid or sex hormones, low mucus, saliva or tear production, or even slowly rising blood sugar levels that are paradoxically seen oftentimes in continuous ketogenic dieters. You can find more on the reasoning behind this in the introduction on the importance of diet (page xv).

A normal meal on the PKDproof program is pretty simple. A little more than three quarters of the plate are taken up with non-starchy, nutrient-rich, organic vegetables that have been steamed or baked, not fried. Almost one quarter of your plate is highly nutrient-dense grass-fed lamb, beef or maybe even pasture-raised pork on some occasions. However, it is wise to prioritize red meat because of its nutrient density and the access of sheep and cattle to pasture.

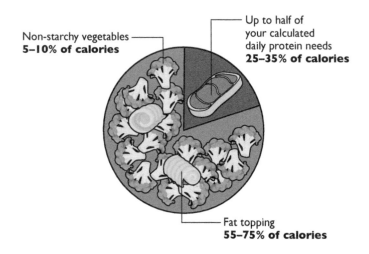

Figure 4: The PKDproof plate

Foods to eat and foods to avoid

The following is a list of foods compiled by author and biohacker Dave Asprey. It represents the best compromise between nutrients and antinutrients. The antinutrients considered in this list are lectins, phytic acid, oxalic acid, phytoestrogens and mold toxins. These anti-nutrients gum up the works in your body, including the kidneys; they steal minerals and create painful and dangerous crystals in the body that can injure surrounding tissues, which has also been discovered to be one of the sources of kidney injury. They can also create inflammation and even be carcinogenic. I discuss them in detail later in this chapter. Nutrient density moves the food towards 'good' while antinutrient and toxin density moves it towards 'bad'.

Table 2: Basics of the PKDproof program: What to eat on the Bulletproof Diet – simplified list. Note that some foods listed are high in oxalates (page 45) that should additionally be taken into account

Beverages	
Good	Filtered water, mineral water, water with lemon/lime, green tea
Medium	Freshly brewed iced tea, fresh nut milk, raw grass-fed A2 milk
Bad	Sodas, sweetened drinks, aspartame drinks, sports drinks
Veggies	
Good	Asparagus, avocado, bok choy, broccoli, Brussels sprouts, cauliflower, celery, cucumber, fennel, olives, cooked kale (high oxalate), cooked collard greens
Medium	Cabbage, lettuce, radishes, summer squash, zucchini, onion, shallots, cilantro, artichokes, butternut squash, green beans, green onion, leeks, parsley
Bad	Eggplant, peas, peppers, spinach (high oxalate), tomatoes, mushrooms, beets (high oxalate), raw collards, raw chard, raw kale (high oxalate), raw spinach (high oxalate), corn (except fresh), canned veggies, soy
Fats	
Good	Coconut oil, pastured egg yolks, grass-fed animal fat, avocado oil, grass-fed butter and ghee, C8 MCT oil
Medium	Palm oil, palm kernel, extra-virgin olive oil (1-2 tbsp/week), pastured bacon fat, C8 and C10 MCT oil
Bad	Duck and goose fat, grain-fed butter and ghee, factory chicken fat, safflower oil, sunflower oil, canola (rapeseed oil), peanut oil, soy, cottonseed oil, corn oil, flaxseed oil

Table 2 (cont'd)

Nuts, seeds and legumes	
Good	Coconut, coconut flour, raw pistachios, cashews, macadamia, walnuts
Medium	Almonds (high oxalate), pecans, sunflower seeds, chestnuts, hazelnuts, roasted pistachios
Bad	sprouted legumes, Brazil nuts, garbanzo beans, hummus, dried peas, most legumes, flaxseed, chia seeds, soy, soy nuts, corn nuts

Protein	
Good	Grass-fed beef and lamb, pastured eggs and gelatin, colostrum, pastured collagen protein, low-mercury wild fish (anchovies, haddock, petrale sole, sardines, sockeye salmon, summer flounder, trout), grass-fed whey protein concentrate
Medium	Pastured pork, clean whey isolate, pastured duck and goose, hemp protein
Bad	Factory-farmed eggs, pastured chicken and turkey, heated whey, factory-farmed meat of any kind, high-mercury or farmed seafood

Dairy	
Good	Organic grass-fed butter and ghee, colostrum
Medium	Grass-fed raw A2 cow's cheese, such as Parmigiano Reggiano, raw sheep and goat cheese, non-organic grass-fed ghee or butter, organic grass-fed cream, grass-fed sheep's yogurt
Bad	Skimmed or low-fat milk, fake butter/'spreads', pasteurized non-organic milk, powdered milk, factory dairy, dairy replacer

Starch/carbs	
Good	Organic acacia, partially-hydrolyzed guar gum (great for gut bacteria as a prebiotic), sweet potato, yam, carrot, raw low-pesticide honey
Medium	Pumpkin, butternut squash, rinsed organic local white rice, cassava, tapioca

Bad	Wheat, corn, millet, other grains, potato starch, corn starch, conventional gluten-free flour, garbanzo flour
Fruit	
Good	Avocado, blackberries, coconut, cranberries, lemon, lime, raspberries (high oxalate)
Medium	Blueberries, pineapple, strawberries, tangerine, grapefruit, pomegranate
Bad	Bananas, dates, grapes, guava, mango, melons, papaya, passion fruit, persimmon, plantain, watermelon
Sweeteners	
Good	Xylitol, erythritol, stevia, monk fruit, d-ribose
Medium	Sorbitol, maltitol, non-GMO dextrose, glucose, raw honey
Bad	White sugar, brown sugar, agave syrup, processed honey, high-fructose corn syrup
Cooking	
Good	Raw or not cooked, lightly heated
Medium	Steamed *al dente*, convection baked or baked at 320°F (160°C) or below, simmered, boiled, poached, lightly grilled, *sous vide*, slow cooked, pressure cooked, air fried
Bad	Burnt, blackened, charred, deep fried, microwaved

Special note on dairy

As it turns out, many people are intolerant of dairy without ever noticing. They might feel fatigued, have rashes or autoimmune issues caused by an intolerance to their never-ending dairy consumption. So please, when you begin the Bulletproof Diet, refrain from dairy except for butter for at least three months. Watch for symptoms for about three days after trying to reintroduce it.

Antinutrients

Now that you know what foods to limit and which foods to enjoy, let's look further at the details of the stuff you will be avoiding this way.

We all learned in school what nutrients are. We need them for optimal bodily function. When we are deficient, we get sick over the long term and all sorts of problems ensue. So, what on earth are antinutrients?

If you look at it from a basic perspective, there are two types of food on the planet – the type that can run away when you're trying to eat it and the type that can't. Since plants have roots, they can't move and so evolutionarily they had to come up with different mechanisms for protecting themselves from being eaten, so that their species could propagate and continue. These mechanisms have evolved to block essential biochemical pathways in their natural predators like bugs, insects and smaller animals. Whenever these antinutrients have a strong negative effect on whatever creature is trying to eat a specific plant, the creature is more likely to avoid eating this plant in the future, improving the chances of survival of the plant species. Often times these antinutrients don't have nearly as strong an effect on us humans as they would on our insect and animal friends, but the effects are still there, especially if you are genetically prone to them. They can be a real issue and lead to chronic health problems without you ever knowing. There are multiple categories of antinutrient and they are probably more plentiful than we can go into in this book. The Bulletproof Diet template does its best to categorize plants from least to most toxic while having the highest possible nutrient content.

Some of the most pervasive antinutrients are lectins, phytic acid, oxalic acid, phytoestrogens, mycotoxins and linoleic acid. Let's look at these next.

Lectins

You have almost certainly heard of gluten. That's one of the most pernicious lectins, found in wheat. And while some lectins can be destroyed through heat, gluten is pretty much impossible to inactivate. While in ancient varieties of wheat, gluten wasn't such a big issue, modern forms of it have been bred to contain even more gluten than they used to.

Lectins are commonly found in many vegetables, the highest levels being in grains, beans, other legumes, and nightshade-family vegetables like potatoes, tomatoes and bell peppers. These are well known for punching little holes in the walls of our digestive tract, binding directly to the gut wall and inhibiting nutrient absorption.

Lectins also feed bacterial strains which produce endotoxin, which is even worse news and a horrible one–two punch, as not only will more unwanted material from the gut end up in the bloodstream, but it will also be higher in endotoxin, putting us at higher risk of injury and cyst growth.

A simple way to inactivate some lectins, for example in legumes, is to soak them overnight, or for 24 hours optimally, and then pressure-cook them. That's the only way I'll consume lentils on rare occasions, and it gives me basically no digestive issues, in contrast to plain cooked lentils.

Phytic acid

This common nutrient-sapping antinutrient is used by plants to bind to minerals, specifically to keep them around as nutrients for their own seeds. When phytic acid binds to minerals, it becomes phytate. The presence of phytic acid can basically invalidate any data on minerals in plant foods, since many minerals are measurably there but not bioavailable. Therefore, these minerals can't really be counted towards nutrient intake and, even worse, excess phytic acid can even bind to additional minerals once inside the body. This way you can actually end up with a net negative effect on minerals when you consume supposed mineral-rich foods that pack a lot of phytic acid.

Historically, it is even possible to see the impact of phytates on human evolution with the dawn of the agricultural age. Height and bone density went down and diseases rose when humans began cultivating staple foods high in phytic acid, like grains and legumes.

Oxalic acid

News about the dangers of oxalic acid has been making the rounds in the kidney world for a couple of years now, which is very fortunate. Word is getting out there that this antinutrient is actually responsible for most kidney stones (calcium oxalate stones). It is also responsible for painful sex in some women, since microscopic stones deposit in the soft tissues of the vagina.

Oxalic acid is mostly found in leafy greens, spinach being the worst offender, containing just about 10 times more than the next worst food. So no, you won't be getting a lot of iron or calcium from your spinach, but you can at least prevent your spinach from taking those precious minerals from you. Have you ever noticed your teeth feeling kind of rough after eating especially raw spinach? That's the oxalic acid binding to the calcium in your teeth.

Now we can use this mechanism to our advantage: the next time you decide to cook spinach, which shouldn't be that often, just add a heaping tablespoon or two of calcium carbonate to the cooking water. That way the oxalic acid will be bound to calcium inside your dish and any phytates, too will be fully bound before you can even ingest them, rendering them unproblematic.

The same technique can be used for all other cooked foods that are high in oxalates. Discarding the cooking water or steaming them also helps a great deal.

It is important to note that the propensity to get kidney stones depends largely on your body's pH, so as long as you're not going overboard with oxalates and you're taking the proper precautions, it's okay to have a moderate amount of them every now and then. However, going all out and trying to avoid all oxalic acid consumption will leave you more likely to consume foods high in the other antinutrients, which is why the balanced approach outlined in the Bulletproof Diet food list was chosen.

Phytoestrogens

Now some plant foods actually don't just inhibit our biology; they also mimic it. Want an example? Enter soybeans! While soybean protein actually has a pretty good amino acid composition (more details on page 64–65 under DIAAS score) – that is, at least compared to all the other plant proteins – sadly, among other antinutrients, these beans also contain phytoestrogens, which mimic human estrogen by binding to estrogen receptors. Now there is still some debate about how much of an issue this really is. One perspective is that phytoestrogens basically give you an estrogen effect, while the other perspective is that they actually block estrogen receptors by sticking to them. Some research, however, is showing reduced sperm quality and a reduction in testosterone. One study[1] even showed that babies fed soy-based formula developed in accordance with exogenous estrogen exposure, meaning their development changed as if they were being given extra estrogen, making them more feminine. In any case, I believe it's not a good idea to have a plant defense mechanism messing around with my hormones one way or the other.

Mycotoxins

Mycotoxins, or mold toxins, are the dangerous stuff that mold emits, especially when it's stressed. They are commonly found in large amounts in wheat, corn, other grains, peanuts, fruit, chocolate and wine. In addition, products from grain-fed animals, like milk or fatty meat, can accumulate mold toxins, as farmers are still allowed to sell their moldy grain as animal feed. This means that foods that seem innocuous might still contain mycotoxins that lead to low-grade inflammation and chronic health issues down the line.

Frequently eating mold, or breathing in its spores when living in a moldy house or driving a moldy car, can wreck your health and lead to asthma, allergies, immune suppression and, over the long term, even cancer, heart disease and kidney damage.[2]

Always choose high-quality, fresh or frozen produce and grains. If you're going to have nuts, avoid any with an 'off' taste and skip peanuts altogether. Don't cut off moldy or mushy parts of foods either; throw affected items away however wasteful that may seem. When you can see the mold, it's already far too late. The notable exception to this rule is avocado – if you do a good job of cutting the mold out, the rest of the avocado is probably going to be fine to eat.

Also spices, often overlooked, are very susceptible to growing mold. Storing spices above steaming pots or near heat sources, as so many of us do, can create the perfect environment for mold to grow. So it's best to store them in a cool, dry place away from heat and steam, and never shake them over the steaming pot. Instead, use a spoon. It's also important to avoid spice mixes containing black pepper, as in addition to its devastating effects on the permeability of our gut lining, it is always contaminated with mold. Opting for individual organic spices gives you better quality and control.

Linoleic acid

Even though you will be limiting this antinutrient using the Bulletproof Diet template, it still bears explaining why linoleic acid is such an important factor to be aware of. Polyunsaturated fatty acids (PUFAs), most notably the omega-6 variants, and even more specifically linoleic acid, are among the worst components in our food today.

While linoleic acid is actually considered an essential fatty acid, over the past 100 years, our intake of it has skyrocketed from a measly 1-3% of all calorie intake to a whopping 15-20%. While the pre-Industrial Revolution levels were biologically adequate, at this much higher level, it becomes a big problem. Particularly prevalent sources in the modern diet would be soy, peanuts and canola (rapeseed) oil, as described below. This increase has had a disastrous effect on the human population as a whole and virtually nobody knows about it. Linoleic acid in excess damages our metabolism and robs our mitochondria of their ability to generate energy, very similar to the effects of injury. You know what this means by now. If energy is not being produced by aerobic respiration (oxygen-using metabolism) inside the mitochondria, the only other option is to use fermentation of glucose or glutamine, which, as we have seen, promotes cyst growth and is the basis for rapid cell proliferation.

This growth-promoting effect of linoleic acid can be observed in cancer, where it upregulates tumor growth,[3] and we can even see it in some research papers on PKD. One study set out to test the impact of dietary PUFAs on PKD by giving rodents different amounts of soy bean oil.[4] Soy bean oil is 55% linoleic acid. An increase in soy bean oil consumption actually increased cyst growth in the test group. As we can see by now, this type of fat does not give the same benefit as we are seeing with biologically aligned ketogenic diets consisting mostly of saturated fat in terms of calories.

By now we can probably assume that the rodents' ability to produce energy in their mitochondria via aerobic respiration was blocked by the high intake of linoleic acid, leading more cells into a mode of fermentation, favoring a low ATP to NAD$^+$ ratio (as explained on page 6) and thereby accelerating cyst growth and cell injury.

Who can say how much cyst growth and mitochondrial injury is triggered by consuming these toxic, often oxidized oils? New research suggests they are responsible for an enormous amount of disease in the general population, including cancer, heart attacks, obesity, sunburn and more. For example, one 2021 study found linoleic acid could induce mitochondrial dysfunction and increase cancer growth by making it harder for the immune system's white blood cells to fight it.[5]

To be safe, a good idea is to cut down linoleic acid intake to something similar to what was available before the food industry started mass-producing vegetable oils. So, about 1-2% of calorie intake.

Common foods high in linoleic acid are vegetable oils like soybean oil, corn oil and sunflower oil as well as processed foods like chips, crackers and baked goods. Additionally, some nuts and seeds are naturally high in it. Of course, margarine and shortening, used in baking and frying, are high in linoleic acid.

In the protein department, conventionally-raised poultry and even pork has elevated levels of linoleic acid from their grain-based feed. Fast-food items, using vegetable oils for frying and cooking, are another source of linoleic acid in the modern diet. However, even good old olive oil still has a considerable amount, which is why for PKD reversal we try to replace it with MCT oil wherever possible; 1-2 tbsp per week is probably okay.

Stearic acid

Following the Bulletproof Diet, you will get a lot more of this in your diet than linoleic acid, and for good reason. You see, mitochondria in PKD cells aren't just extremely underused, they are also, in part, broken.

In a 2020 study, Italian researchers examined in detail the mitochondria of a mouse model of PKD. What they noticed were several alterations 'including reduced mitochondrial mass, altered structure and fragmentation'. Also, they found reduced expression of the proteins responsible for mitochondrial fusion, fusion being the process by which the fragmentation can be rescued.[6] So, to put it bluntly, mitochondria in cells expressing the PKD mutation are broken into smaller pieces, and the pieces themselves also don't quite look like they should, which in biology means they also don't work as they should. In cell biology, structure equals function. So, one question we might ask is, how can we mend these broken mitochondria, or how can we induce mitochondrial fusion?

One very interesting way to induce mitochondrial fusion is the consumption of stearic acid.[7] What is stearic acid? It's about 10% of butter, 25-30% of suet and up to 35% of cocoa butter. It's also used in soap and candles. Basically, it is one of the main constituents of healthy dietary saturated fats. Think of it as the anti-linoleic acid.

Some great ways to get it include tallow (use it in cooking) and cocoa butter (use it in desserts and / or bulletproof coffee). You can even get stearic acid-enhanced butter oil online.

The omega-6 to omega-3 ratio

Now that we've talked about the most insidious of the omega-6 fats, it's also important to address the overall balance between omega-6 and omega-3 essential fatty acids in the body. Actually, our intake of omega-3 fatty acids is hypothesized to be one of the reasons that we now are able to maintain such big brains. After all, 50% of the fat content of our brains is made up of omega-3. And while we used to get lots of omega-3 from eating fish and, yes, actual brains from big ruminant animals, nowadays many people don't eat fish at all, and the vast majority of course have never eaten brains once in their life. You see, humans are at a disadvantage here. While big ruminant animals have the ability to convert plant-based omega-3 fats from all kinds of grasses, leaves and herbs to their bioavailable forms EPA and DHA, humans are so bad at this process that even in the best case scenario it's just up to 5%.[8] So really, if we want to have a good intake of omega-3 fatty acids, it needs to come from animal foods. Optimally that's wild 'SMASH' fish, which are lower in heavy metals (salmon, mackerel, anchovies, sardines and herring), foods like wild salmon roe (even lower in heavy metals) or a fish oil or algae oil supplement. Yes, of course you can also eat brains if you can get them in your country; just be safe about the preparation. There are some concerns about disease transmission. Some companies offer a freeze-dried extract in capsule form.

A low omega-6 to omega-3 ratio, at about 4:1 to 1:1, is therefore optimal for body functions, evolutionarily consistent and also – as described later – correlates with lower blood pressure. This all-important ratio is jeopardized even more by most people's high intake of omega-6 fatty acids from processed plant oils as described above. Avoid these at all costs.

As mentioned already, another source of omega-6 fats is nuts. Note that these will contain better quality fats if the nuts are raw rather than processed. The lowest omega-6-to omega-3 ratio nuts are macadamias (4:1) and walnuts (6:1). The worst offenders are peanuts at a whopping 1720:1. Avoid. (They're also routinely moldy, as I've said.) Keep in mind however, that omega-3 fat from nuts comes in the form of alpha-linolenic acid, or ALA, which is converted to biologically active omega-3 in the form of DHA or EPA at a rate of 0.5-5% depending on your intake of omega-6, as omega-6 competes with ALA for the same enzyme, so for most people it's on the low end of the scale. This means that the omega-3 in plant foods is not as relevant for your own omega-3 intake as you might assume.

In the next chapter we will look at the practicalities of following the PKDproof program.

Chapter 5

How to do the PKDproof program right

About food quality and cost

These days money has gotten tighter for most of the population. This means it's very understandable people would look for ways to save money, and one very obvious way would be to save on food. This is actually not a bad idea. Some really good ways to do this are:

- Fasting
- Skipping processed foods
- Skipping restaurant meals
- Buying in bulk
- Buying frozen foods.

Now, what is *not* a good way to save on food is to lower food quality. You see, you can regard the higher price we pay for organic foods as the base price. A conventionally grown vegetable, for example, will be discounted from that base price because it contains some extra poison. If you look at it rationally, at the current state of our food system, most foods are laden with herbicides, pesticides, heavy metals and other toxic materials.

If the manufacturer can get you to buy it, you're getting a discount. But you're paying with your health. Of course, organic foods are far from perfect; grains especially tend to contain some residue of glyphosate (Roundup) even when you buy organic. Luckily, I do not recommend you eat grains at all, so we can dodge that bullet.

For buying vegetables, if money is tight, there is a list called the 'clean 15' that is updated every year by the US-based 'environmental working group' (www.ewg.org). This list contains the vegetables that have the lowest amounts of toxic chemicals even when produced conventionally. This is helpful not only in saving money, but also because the availability of organic vegetables is often limited. Getting frozen vegetables can be a good option too.

Special caution is warranted for avocados: if you buy conventionally grown varieties, do not touch the skin with your bare hands; instead, use a paper or plastic bag as a glove and scrub the outside with dishwashing liquid at home. The pesticides may not make it all the way to the inside, but even touching them is bad news.

Regarding your meat options, there is a similar story. Of course, it can be cheaper to just buy any old factory-farmed ground (minced) beef or pork or chicken and use that to get in your daily protein. But these animals usually have been severely mistreated, which not only is horrible for them and the environment, but is also horrible for anyone eating their meat. You see, animals store toxins in their fat tissue, just like we do. Any toxins they consume during their lifetime accumulate to some degree in their fat. This means that whenever you're stuck in some food desert and your only option is to have factory-farmed meat, the leanest cuts will be your best choice. Also, eating beef instead of chicken or pork will be a better choice because cattle actually have the capacity to convert any fat they eat to saturated fat, meaning at least the fat profile of the small amount of fat you're going to eat will be far superior to pork or chicken, which always mirrors the fat profile of whatever they ate during their lifetimes.

But of course the much better option is to stock up your freezer with high-quality grass-fed and grass-finished beef or lamb. Being grass-finished is super-important because a lifetime of grass-feeding can be virtually nullified by a final grain feeding phase that many producers have their cattle go through right before slaughter. So make sure you are getting grass-fed *and* grass-finished beef. Ground (minced) beef can be very cost effective, easy to prepare and also very space saving when you're trying to buy in bulk and put it in the freezer. Establishing a connection with a local beef farmer can yield bulk discounts and, even more importantly, ensure your beef is actually grass-fed and grass-finished. Knowing your producer is always best. There are also good mail-order options for grass-fed beef online. A great way to make sure you are getting grass-fed, grass-finished beef is to find a farmer that has heritage breeds like Galloway. These breeds can't have grains at all. Another good way to source meat is to go by source country. Irish beef and lamb is usually grass-fed, as is Australian or New Zealand beef or lamb.

Important note: To save money on cooking fats, like butter, you can ask your local farmer or butcher to sell you some beef trimmings. Maybe they will even give it to you for free. You can use these to render your own tallow for cooking. Just find a slow-cooker, fill it with beef trimmings and leave it running for about 15 to 24 hours on the low setting. Stir every once in a while until the fat stops sizzling. Only use wooden or metal tools inside, as plastic can deform and even melt very quickly in hot fat like this. Doing this can save you a lot of money for cooking, and you'll be getting a lot of nutrients in the process.

Bulletproof coffee

On the PKDproof program, you can still get a great start to your day, even though you might choose to have your fasting window in the morning. How does that work? Enter bulletproof coffee. This is one of the main staples of the PKDproof program. As a mainstay of the Bulletproof Diet, it's an amazing way to get focus and energy, as well as some extra ketones, while getting most of the cell-recycling effects of intermittent fasting. So this is our ticket to do it effortlessly, without feeling hungry. You can find a detailed recipe on page 219, but suffice it to say, the main ingredients are mold-free coffee (so you don't injure your kidneys), C8 MCT oil (gives you extra ketones) and grass-fed butter (emulsifies the mixture and adds some nice nutrients). Blend it up and there's what feels like breakfast – but it's not, as it's not actually breaking your fast, at least not in regards to the mechanisms we are most interested in.

Bulletproof coffee: the benefits

As you're going to consume this quite a lot in your morning routine, it's important you use the right ingredients and preparation methods when making bulletproof coffee. The oils in coffee — kahweol and cafestol — act as powerful anti-inflammatory agents that shield against oxidative stress and DNA damage, which is a main issue in PKD. Preserving these oils by using brewing methods like a French press or an espresso machine (aluminum-free) is a good idea as paper filters remove them from the coffee.

Moreover, to optimize the health benefits, it's vital to blend the butter and MCT oil into the coffee on high power. This process transforms the butter into micelles, which are basically tiny water-soluble droplets of fat. This helps a lot with the body's utilization of this fat for energy. Consuming butter without blending it with the coffee won't yield the same beneficial results. Find a high-powered glass blender without plastic parts on the inside. Be sure to check the bottom, too, as cheaper blenders often come with bottom inside plates made of plastic or aluminum. You want glass and stainless steel only. This is important as you are looking at using this device daily, with hot and acidic liquid that is prone to dissolve plastic or oxidize and dissolve aluminum to potentially poison you in the long term.

The cheap approach to this is a stainless-steel stick blender in a big glass jar, preferably with a square footprint, as otherwise it will quickly splash out of the jar.

Bulletproof coffee: why it works

1. Bulletproof coffee makes it very easy to stick to the fasting window of 16-18 hours, since it will easily make you feel full for a really long time. These will be the only calories that are allowed inside the fasting window.

2. The second advantage is a substantial increase in ketones due to the MCT oil, as well as the coffee itself, which doubles ketone production and also inhibits mTOR. A double win.

3. The third advantage is, that by blending the fat with the coffee you create millions of little micelles that make it a lot easier for your body to metabolize the fats that are in the coffee.

4. Blending the coffee for 30 seconds structures the water by putting it through the vortex that results from blending. Some research suggests that the water itself becomes more available to the body that way.[1]

5. Fat intake is actually the largest endogenous (meaning the body's own) stimulator for somatostatin production. Pharmaceutical analogues of somatostatin, like octreotide, have been shown to limit growth of total kidney volume in PKD significantly. In addition, the increased uptake of fatty acids also possibly raises the amount of intracellular calcium (Ca^{2+}), which is low in PKD.

6. The water surrounding the fat micelles is actually

'fourth phase water', also called 'EZ water'. There has been groundbreaking research by Dr Gerald Pollack at the University of Washington that shows this form of water is the most accessible cellular water.[1]

7. MCT oil has been shown to greatly reduce the damage done by endotoxin in the gut. That is another reason why I add MCT oil to all my meals. This is especially helpful when you also have liver cysts because MCT oil is metabolized directly in the liver.

8. Grass-fed butter gives you a nice bump of highly bioavailable fat-soluble vitamins.

It is not entirely clear if all the effects of pure intermittent fasting remain in place when you consume bulletproof coffee in the morning. However, my personal results have been achieved by incorporating intermittent fasting with this morning drink almost every day. So even if some of the physiology of fasting changes when you consume it, the benefits listed above might just mean it's even more effective for PKD than pure fasting, even though we probably won't see a study on this anytime soon. In the end, it's all about consistency. This breakfast replacement makes it effortless to skip eating until lunchtime. If you like, you can integrate some days of pure intermittent fasting for good measure, whenever you feel that you don't need to have calories. Don't force it. For me, after a couple of years there were many mornings when I did not feel like I needed food. When my body wants it, I have it. When it doesn't, I might not have it. Or you can choose to just have your mold-free coffee black. It totally depends on what you feel like, once you get adapted to the state of ketosis.

Ketosis

Trying to reverse PKD without being in ketosis, reliably and primarily, is like trying to reverse your car without putting it into reverse gear. It just won't happen. All the supplements we might take – possibly with the exception of exogenous ketone supplements – will make it easier to reverse, but they won't do it by themselves.

Regarding exogenous ketone supplements (like ketone salts or ketone esters), the jury is still out, but any effect they do have is going to be short-lived, and therefore difficult to sustain. For now, it is paramount you make sure to get into, and stay in, ketosis for most of the week. This means you need to keep track of your diet, especially carbohydrate intake, very diligently, especially in the beginning weeks and months. It is very easy to overeat carbohydrates without really noticing. Most people eat a high-carb diet, so what might feel 'low-carb' to them might still be way too high to get into ketosis.

As you're aware now, once PKD cells are doubly mutated (see page 1) – that is, once the second 'hit' has struck them – not much time will pass until their mitochondria get damaged and they go into unlimited proliferation mode and there is no turning back as long as they get their preferred fuels, glucose and glutamine. Our only way to get them to stop proliferating uncontrollably is to restrict their access to these fuels. And because we can't just deprive our body of glucose and glutamine entirely without dying, the next best thing is to switch it over to fat and ketones as an alternative fuel source, which already takes care of the glucose part of the equation, and can be sufficient for many people.

To recap, ketones and even the fats they are made from are always metabolized with oxygen, yielding a lot more energy and therefore lasting for a lot longer than glucose or glutamine metabolized through aerobic glycolysis or glutaminolysis. Either the cell metabolizes ketones with oxygen and thereby stops or even reverses its proliferation, or it dies. We don't know exactly which of these scenarios is more likely to happen or happens more often, but both work in our favor.

If carbohydrates in the diet are higher than 40 or 50 grams of net carbs per day (meaning carbs minus fiber and/or sugar alcohols like xylitol or erythritol), most people will still be able to produce enough glucose from those carbohydrates to run on as fuel and consequently won't reach the threshold for ketosis. When you do reach that threshold, and you are in a ketogenic state for some time, you should feel absolutely fine, or even better than on a carbohydrate-rich diet.

If you get any specific ailments when you're in ketosis, you're likely not fully adapted yet, or sodium deficient so give it a couple of weeks and use salt liberally. If it's been longer than that, it might be a good opportunity to look closer and find out what is blocking your adaptation or missing from your diet. More on that in Chapter 12, Common pitfalls.

One often overlooked aspect of ketogenic dieting is the influence of our body's oxaloacetate levels on our ability to produce ketones. These stores get replenished whenever we eat protein or carbohydrates. Now when we are fat-adapted after several months on a ketogenic diet, our body will be able to directly metabolize fatty acids in the mitochondrial citric acid cycle to produce energy, even bypassing the need for ketone production. This ability may get more and more efficient the longer we are on a high-fat diet. The more efficient our body becomes at this process, the more difficult it may become to achieve high levels of blood ketones. This is the normal progression of metabolic adaptation and can be different in different people. However, this process of direct oxidation of fatty acids for energy is dependent on sufficient oxaloacetate levels. If your goal is to achieve higher ketone levels for therapeutic benefit, which we don't know is necessary, you can deplete your oxaloacetate stores more quickly by decreasing the sources of oxaloacetate (protein and carbohydrates) and/or increasing fat intake.

Fat to protein-and-carbohydrate ratios starting at 1.5:1 and going up to 4:1 can be necessary if higher levels of ketones are desired to speed up the healing process. 2:1 is a common ratio used in metabolic therapy for cancer.[2]

Keep in mind that protein is an essential nutrient and should not fall below your minimum requirements for extended periods of time. If you need high ratios to obtain significant levels of ketosis and cannot consume your required amount of protein that way, you can cycle and have some extra protein on the other days.

Doing high fat-to-protein ratio days back-to-back is more efficient than spacing them out over the week. Fasting and exogenous ketone supplements are other ways to achieve higher ketone levels. There is more on that in Chapter 12 on 'Common pitfalls' on page 181.

Demystifying protein

So, protein, right? Everybody in the kidney world keeps talking about it and many are even afraid of it. The fact of the matter is, protein is the most fundamental building block of our bodies. Molecularly, proteins are actually literal tiny machines doing physical work. For example, a small motor protein called kinesin actually looks like a little man walking a rope, carrying a big bag on his head (see Figure 5). Really, it's fascinating. I highly recommend doing an online search for 'kinesin walking' and looking at some of the animations.

Another example to look at is the recently decoded protein TRPV5, which lines the intestines and kidneys and acts as a gate to increase or decrease the influx of calcium, depending on the availability of calcium-sensing proteins.

It is not crucially important to understand what these proteins are doing in detail; this just goes to show that protein is much more than something needed for bodybuilders. Proteins quite literally are the micro-machines in our bodies and without them we cannot function. So this leads us to the common myth that somehow chronic protein restriction could be a good idea in kidney disease.

Why should protein restriction be considered a good thing in PKD?

Whenever amino acids from protein that we eat undergo a process called 'deamination', which is the removal of nitrogen from the amino acids by an enzyme, extra nitrogen is produced that our kidneys need to get rid of. This is usually not a problem, but in later stages of kidney disease, there can be a build-up of nitrogen which is expressed in an elevated level of blood urea nitrogen (BUN) on a blood test. Whenever you see an elevated level of BUN on your results, you might want to consider replacing part of your protein with essential amino acids; there is more on that on page 75. You do not want to *reduce* protein intake unless it exceeds your daily needs. It might make sense, however, to keep protein at around 25 g per meal and space it out as much as possible to give your kidneys time to process the accumulated nitrogen.

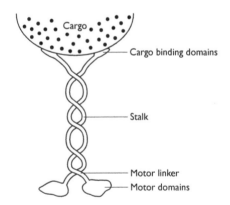

Figure 5: Kinesin – a great example of how fascinating our bodies' little machines called proteins really are. Just like a delivery truck on a highway, this motor protein ensures that vital materials are transported to cells that need them.

Protein restriction, while having been a popular recommendation amongst nephrologists for many decades, is still contested as an intervention in PKD and other chronic kidney diseases. Its effect on slowing the speed of decline is actually quite small, only reducing the rate of decline in eGFR by 0.53 ml/min/year in one study, while not clearly reducing overall mortality (meaning protein restrictors just die of something else, but not later).[3] This is, because protein intake itself does not negatively affect kidney function. On the contrary, higher protein intakes, especially of animal protein, lead to higher kidney function. How does this work?

To be clear, the current scientific understanding is that nephrons, being the functional units of the kidney, cannot regenerate or be regrown once damaged or lost. However, the glomeruli, which form the head of the nephrons and are responsible for filtering the blood, can actually increase in volume. This is known as glomerular hypertrophy and can compensate for lost kidney function. This is the main mechanism by which we can regain kidney function according to the current state of the science, and it is of course dependent on adequate protein intake.

Many nephrologists still believe that somehow this is a problem, being under the impression that more function now leads to less function later. Sort of a wear-and-tear paradigm. This hypothesis is what led to the widespread recommendation of low-protein diets, which haven't been able to prolong the time to kidney failure in human studies.[4]

As quoted in a 2022 study entitled 'Protein Restriction for CKD: Time to Move On', the pioneer of hemodialysis, F Parsons said: 'All a low protein diet does is to shrink the patient down to the size of his kidneys.'[5]

So if we can increase kidney function with protein, what's the catch? A 2021 study tried to come up with a threshold of how much glomerular hypertrophy (growth of glomeruli) was safe without scarring occurring.[6] The study found that when the maximum diameter of these glomeruli exceeds a certain threshold (224 μm in this study), scarring becomes increasingly likely.

So there is a limit to how much the glomeruli can compensate before the process leads to structural damage. Staying within the compensatory range (below the threshold of 224 μm) does not necessarily lead to scarring. This indicates that there is a safe range of hypertrophy where the glomeruli can enlarge to enhance their function.

Unfortunately, getting your maximal glomerular diameter measured is still reserved for research settings. For now, a good indicator that we're in the compensatory range might be protein in urine decreasing or staying the same while eGFR increases. Of course, this can result in a false positive when protein intake is increased. It should also be noted that there is some evidence suggesting these compensatory changes mainly work using animal protein, while plant proteins block this ability.[7] So, just as adequate protein intake is crucial to maintain good kidney function and even enable compensatory mechanisms, extreme protein restriction leads to a faster decline in function. In consequence, if your BUN (blood urea nitrogen – see page 73) levels are normal and you're not in PKD stage 4 or worse, you should make sure you are consuming adequate levels of high-quality protein. In fact, even if you are stage 4 or worse, you still need adequate protein intake, but you can replace part of it with essential amino acids. More on that on page 75.

Now what do I mean by high-quality? When considering protein quality, you need to think of the composition of amino acids (the basic elements that make up all proteins), their bioavailability and the antinutrients that might come with them. To help us gauge this, there is something called the DIAAS score. It describes how bioavailable proteins actually are, based on their amino acid composition. As you can see from Figure 6, even the best plant protein scores worse than the worst animal protein.

In addition, plant proteins often come packaged with a hefty load of antinutrients like lectins, phytates, oxalates and

Animal protein sources

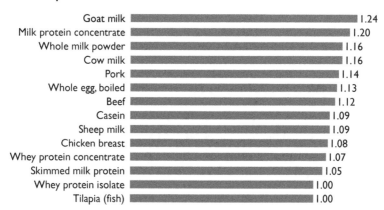

Plant protein sources

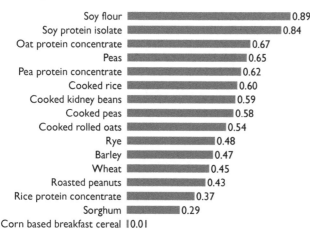

Figure 6: DIAAS (digestible indispensable amino acid) score for a range of foods indicating relative protein quality

phytoestrogens that can wreak all sorts of havoc in our bodies by inhibiting important processes, gumming up the works, disrupting hormone function and robbing us of essential minerals. Also, all unprocessed plant-protein sources are high in carbohydrates and therefore not a good fit for our program. The safest plant proteins are listed in the Bulletproof Diet food list (see page 39).

If you are vegetarian or vegan for ethical reasons, please refer to the section in Chapter 7 (see page 93).

Calculating protein needs

For optimal bodily function, the current scientific estimate is that we need somewhere around 1.3 to 1.8 grams of protein per kilogram of optimal body weight for proper muscle building.[8] Mind you, muscle mass is one of the most important factors for longevity, especially in old age.

Therefore, if you are overweight, you can use a BMI calculator to find your optimal body weight and then use that as a basis for this calculation. If you have a lot of muscle, you can go towards the high end of the range, but then again you probably already have a regimen that works for you.

You can find my calculator for body weight, BMI and protein needs at: www.ReversingPKD.com/report

Bad proteins

So, we talked about the need for grass-fed meats before. You might be asking yourself: 'What's the issue with regular beef? Or even organically raised beef?' Conventional, or even organic, meats are not in the 'good' category of the Bulletproof Diet since the cattle are still being fed grains, albeit organically grown ones, which in turn cause inflammation in their bodies.

Did you know, cows naturally cannot even digest grains?

When a calf is transitioned to grains too quickly, there's something called grain poisoning and it can be deadly to the young cow. To combat this issue, cows are inoculated with a yeast infection in their rumen that aids the fermentation of grains. Of course, this yeast infection is not without consequences and leads to inflammation and constant flatulence. Grass-fed cattle might produce less methane out of the gate[9] and might even be carbon negative, offsetting CO_2 production on a large scale. Grass-grazing and grain-fed cows emit comparable levels of methane due to the nature of the cow's digestive system; however, grazing keeps grassland in a rapid growth phase, sequestering way more carbon in the soil than they actually emit.[10]

When you eat a conventionally fed animal, some of the inflammatory messenger molecules, yeasts and grain-derived pesticides like glyphosate that circulate in their tissues will end up in your food, and therefore in your body. This in turn can only contribute to cyst growth. And if that wasn't enough, consuming conventionally raised meats can also expose you to the risk of urinary tract infections (UTIs) due to potential contamination with *E. coli* bacteria. Recent research has highlighted that contaminated meats are a main source of *E. coli* responsible for UTIs in humans, chicken being the worst offender.[11]

So there is no room for negotiation on these kinds of meat or even fish. Even if you think having fish at the restaurant is the healthy option, think again. Farmed salmon has been shown to contain up to four times as many toxic PCBs (polychlorinated biphenyls, which are persistent, cancer-causing chemicals) as mass-produced beef.[12] You can get away with cheap eggs from time to time since they seem to be pretty protected from the toxic environment most chickens grow up in. Wild salmon, especially sockeye, also is a good option. Bigger fish like tuna are full of mercury and therefore bad news for the kidneys and other organs.

When, why and how to eat carbs

While we are doing everything we can to skip starchy foods on ketogenic diet days, there are those days where we need to refuel (see Figure 8). Now, after reading everything about carbohydrates so far, you might feel inclined to skip them altogether and just deal with it; it's all for your health, right?

However, there are of course other aspects to diet that need to be considered. Adequate carbohydrate intake is important for long-term hormonal health in men and women; a long-term ketogenic diet without carbohydrate refeeds has been correlated with lower production of male and female sex hormones, thyroid hormone and even mucus, tears and saliva.

A chronically low carbohydrate intake also, in some people, leads to slowly but steadily increasing blood sugar levels, even when fasted. This of course is not great news for PKD. To prevent this from happening, it is important to intermittently include carbohydrates in the diet. I recommend doing this by simply replacing your usual vegetable intake with starchy vegetables like sweet potatoes, rinsed organic white rice or fruit on this day. Remember to cook with, and discard, excess cooking water for white rice to lower the concentration of dissolved toxins. Of course, there are a lot of other options on the food list; these are just some examples.

You can keep the rest of the diet the same if you like, or you can make some replacements for some beloved high-carb baked goods using alternative flours such as tapioca or rice flour.

Usually women tend to need more carbohydrates than men: one re-feed day per week for men and two re-feed days per week for women might be a good starting point, but your mileage may vary (a lot). Keep a close eye on how you feel regarding energy, sex drive and zest for life when you embark on this program and, if you are adapted to ketosis and you are doing re-feeds but suspect hormones might be declining, this is a good time to get hormones checked and possibly increase carb re-feeds. After all, hormonal health is super-important for the health of the whole body, and the kidneys are no exception to this rule. You need to build a strong foundation first.

Cheat days

On the PKDproof program, we do not plan for cheat days. Let me repeat that: we don't plan for cheat days. Life will give you plenty of moments with limited PKDproof options. Don't sweat it when you are at that wedding or birthday party, just find whatever food fits the program best in that scenario, bring some charcoal capsules and enjoy yourself. The point is, don't schedule cheat days on purpose. Trust me, you will feel much better and stop constantly thinking about the next cheat day like I did. Instead, you will regularly enjoy awesome delicious PKDproof meals and desserts that will not leave you wanting more.

In all seriousness, regularly consuming foods that trigger inflammation in your body is just about the worst thing that you could do to your already burdened kidneys.

Just imagine you were to step on a nail. Once a week. Every week. Just once. How well do you think that wound would heal? It would never even get a chance to improve; rather, it would get nasty and infected. The same goes for cheating on your diet regularly. It will constantly negate the benefits of your progress. For example, your gut takes about one week to heal from a gluten 'attack'. If you do that every week, you are not going to improve much over time.

Your kidneys aren't even in a good place to begin with, since you have this genetic defect. So throwing some inflammation-promoting grains, sweets, bad oils, fried foods, pesticide-laden foods, mass-produced meats or other rubbish their way will go a long way to destroying any kind of healing you might have gotten done throughout the rest of the week. 'But Felix,' you say,

'I need something sweet as a snack to not go crazy!' That's not a problem. There are many healthy options for desserts and other delicious foods in the 'good' category on the Bulletproof Diet.

You can bake delicious desserts with coconut flour and erythritol (a low-calorie, low-carb sugar alcohol) and you can make an awesome pudding using avocado or coconut milk and some gelatin as well as some vanilla powder and other sweeteners like monk fruit or stevia. There are many options and you can enjoy those, even regularly if you wish. I certainly love a sweet dessert, and I don't have to feel guilty about it.

Erythritol has faced some negative media coverage after a 2022 study attempted to link elevated blood levels of erythritol to heart disease. However, the study did not involve subjects *consuming* erythritol. The participants with higher risks had elevated erythritol blood levels, which is a compensatory mechanism and marker for insulin resistance, which is the most likely culprit. Eating erythritol is not associated with these issues.[13]

Water intake

Drinking a lot of water has long been standard medical advice for patients with PKD, the working theory behind this being that high water intake lowers urine osmolality, meaning fewer dissolved particles, which in turn should lower cyclic AMP (cAMP), which is one of the pathways implicated in PKD. The purported benefits of high water intake on improvement of function even go so far as to lead to a serious criticism in the initial trial for tolvaptan, which is the only drug approved for PKD. After the trial was published,[14] the journal in which it appeared published a letter to the editor pointing out the serious design flaw in the study, which was the lack of a placebo group with the same water intake as the treatment group.[15]

However, convincing evidence for a clear benefit of high

water intake in humans with PKD is scarce. Early evidence from animal trials that hinted at a benefit of high water intake was not mirrored in a 2022 study in humans, which compared two treatment arms over the course of three years – one with normal water intake and one with higher water intake at an increase of 0.6-0.75 liters over the control group.[16] Granted, this was not an impressive increase and pales in comparison with the doubling or tripling of water intake for patients starting on tolvaptan. Additional trials investigating higher water intakes have been announced, completed but not yet published. The 'DRINK' trial was completed in 2018 and still never published. We can only speculate as to the reasons for this. One trial that was published recently reported positive results, indicating high water intake correlated with a one-third reduction in the speed of cyst growth.[17]

In any case, when it comes to water intake, you should definitely drink enough, just like anyone should. After all, the kidneys need enough fluid to work with. Is it possible that higher water intakes slow PKD progression? Yes. Do our current human trials look like they do? Possibly.

Don't force yourself to drink ridiculous amounts of water each day, but do make sure you drink enough since, especially with increasing age, people tend to drink too little and that would definitely cause problems. Drinking too much can also cause problems, especially in regard to electrolytes. So, if you choose to drink more water, also make sure to consume higher amounts of electrolytes and test those regularly at your doctor's visits. If you get any cramps, that's your hint that your electrolytes are low. In that case, look first to magnesium and sodium, but potassium deficiency could also be the culprit. It's good to shoot for pale yellow urine color, not dark, but also not colorless. This is the best gauge we have for hydration for now.

If you have problems drinking adequate amounts of water, my recommendation for getting the most water in is to get a large drinking glass and carafe. Small glasses make it look like you have drunk a lot when you really haven't. Large glasses do the opposite. Have it sitting beside you while you work at all times. Just get used to taking a sip every couple of minutes and it makes it really easy to drink 3-4 liters per day.

In addition, when you get up in the morning, make it a rule to immediately down half a liter of water and take half your daily dose of magnesium, maybe with a tablespoon of apple cider vinegar or lemon juice. This always gives me a great head start. This way, by the time you've had your bulletproof coffee, you'll already be up to just about 1 liter.

'But in my case this kind of diet doesn't work,' I hear you say. 'My doctor restricts my intake of certain things and therefore I cannot adhere to this program.' If this sounds like you, proceed to the next chapter.

Chapter 6

Adjustments for low kidney function

What if your doctor says you need to restrict certain nutrients or that keto is not for you? Well, ask them why they want to make these changes. I have listed here some of the lab values that can become elevated in later stages of PKD and which adjustments to the diet make sense in these cases.

BUN (blood urea nitrogen)

An elevated BUN level basically means your body isn't excreting enough of the waste contained within proteins from your diet, or from muscle breakdown for that matter. All the protein we eat, regardless of its source, contains a nitrogen component in its amino acids. As protein is an essential building block for life, you might've noticed that it is not as simple as just restricting it to reduce nitrogen. If you restrict protein, you will lower your BUN, but you might also become protein deficient.

At the risk of repeating what was explained in the previous Chapter, protein deficiency actually seems to be a risk factor for more rapid decline in kidney function as well as muscle loss. This would make sense, right? If you're missing the raw materials, you can't build body parts very well. So you can see why this is a real catch-22 when doctors suggest you restrict protein because of elevated BUN levels. In the long term, especially with old age, this increases the risk for cachexia, which is the scientific term for muscle loss that can often occur later in life.

And there's more to consider. It's not just about lowering the burden that your kidneys have to process; you also need to provide your body with the raw materials that it needs to repair itself in its constant process of cell turnover. The average time it takes to replace every cell in your body is roughly seven to 10 years. Kidney cells too have some limited capability to repair, but this is in part dependent on proper availability of nutrients, including adequate protein. After all, cells need protein to function, acting as enzymes, structural components, signaling molecules and transporters.

Now of course you should not be eating excessive protein. If you are eating more than you need, you can safely cut back. While protein needs vary widely among people with different genetic makeups and different goals, I tend to err on the lower end of the range recommended for muscle building at around 0.6 grams per pound of optimal body weight per day, or 1.3 grams per kilogram, so as to not over-activate mTOR but still allow for decent muscle building. If you are already consuming a similar amount, there is an option to lower nitrogen intake from protein by replacing part of your protein with essential amino acids (see next).

So, now that even the possibly outdated recommendation of restricting protein in the later stages of kidney disease is being revised, what could be a better solution in order to lower the burden on kidney cells while still getting optimal nourishment and enough raw materials?

Exercise can actually lower BUN by preventing deamination of some amino acids as they are incorporated into muscle directly without excess nitrogen. What else?

EAAs and KAEAAs

Replacing part of protein intake with essential amino acid (EAA) powders can be a straightforward and cost-effective way to reduce elevated BUN levels. That way we can reduce nitrogen intake while simultaneously improving absorption. About 50% of the amino acids in proteins we eat are non-essential, meaning our bodies can synthesize them. The other half we definitely need to consume. So getting just the essential amino acids we really need can be a good way to reduce protein and nitrogen intake without going into protein deficiency. To a certain extent this means we can count EAAs roughly double when replacing regular protein.

A 155-pound (70 kg) human would usually consume about 93 grams (g) of protein per day according to our formula. If they decide to replace 40 g of their daily protein intake with EAA powders, they would need approximately 18 g of powder.

Protein contains about 16% nitrogen by weight. Now let's calculate the nitrogen savings:

- 40 g of protein would contribute approximately 6.4 g of nitrogen (16% of 40 g / 40 g).
- As the nitrogen content in EAAs is the same, 18 g EAA powder would contribute approximately 2.88 g of nitrogen (16% of 18 g / 18 g).

By replacing 40 g of protein with 18 g of EAA powder, the person would be reducing their nitrogen intake by 3.52 g for that portion of their diet, bringing the total nitrogen intake for the day to approximately 11.36 g (14.88 g minus 3.52 g), a reduction of about 23.7%.

Now if you want to reduce nitrogen even more, you can use ketoanalogs of these essential amino acids (KAEAAs). Comparatively, using these instead would lead to an even more substantial nitrogen reduction – for example, 'Ketosteril', one of the most prominent KAEAA products, has about 6% nitrogen content due to its modified structure. This would reduce the daily nitrogen intake by 5.32 g, giving a 36% nitrogen reduction without inducing protein deficiency.

However, the choice between EAAs and KAEAAs is not just about nitrogen content. KAEAAs offset the nitrogen with a higher calcium content, which can be a concern for some patients too. Therefore, the choice between using EAAs and KAEAAs depends on your BUN and calcium blood test results, and probably your vitamin D and vitamin K2 status too, as these vitamins mobilize calcium.

EAAs are much cheaper and more widely available, even in a pure form with no additives. KAEAA products usually come in tablet form with lots of additives. This makes EAA powders a more user-friendly and budget-conscious option for those beginning to want to reduce nitrogen.

Research on KAEAAs' impact on kidney function

In a 2018 study, researchers compared a low-protein diet at about 0.27 grams of protein per pound of body weight to a low-protein diet supplemented with ketoanalogs of essential amino acids (KAEAAs). What they found was very interesting: the group on the low-protein diet without additional amino acid supplements went from an average GFR (glomerular filtration rate) of 34 to 26.2 over the course of 14 months. That is an almost 24% loss of kidney function. In contrast, the intervention group supplemented with KAEAAs went from 34.7 to 31.3, just a 10% loss.[1] This shows us that protein restriction as it is still practiced in many doctor's offices to this day, at around 0.3 grams of protein per pound of body weight or less, could be considered a form of malnutrition. So it looks like in part the reason for the decline in kidney function in the study was induced by protein deficiency. This leads us to the conclusion that whenever nitrogen restriction is necessary, KAEAAs or at the very least

EAAs should be used to make up for the difference in amino acid intake. In this study, only a single dosage regimen at 0.045 grams per pound of body weight was tested, which should equate to about 0.1 grams of extra protein per pound of body weight, making study participants still only barely reach the equivalent of 0.4 grams, still far below our recommendation of 0.6 grams of protein per pound of body weight per day.

So you can get EAAs or KAEAAs over-the-counter or you can work with your doctor to get a prescription for KAEAAs. Unflavored EAAs are available at bodybuilding websites, 'Ketorena' offers an over-the-counter KAEAA supplement and prescription forms include 'Ketosteril' and others. Ketoanalogs have been studied at various dosages and are very safe, with the exception of possible elevated calcium levels. If you can, skip the additives by opting for a powdered product. Offset the taste with lemon juice and stevia drops if necessary.

When starting on ketoanalogs, the manufacturer of Ketorena suggests you regularly monitor the following blood levels monthly for three months:

- BUN (blood urea nitrogen)
- Electrolytes
- Calcium
- Phosphate
- PTH
- Creatinine
- Creatinine clearance
- Acid-base balance
- Bicarbonate
- Blood count
- Hemoglobin
- Lipids
- Glycemia
- Transferrin.

Calcium: If you see calcium going out of range, it's probably time to dial back on your vitamin D intake; however, you don't want it to go below 60 ng/dl. If this is not enough, dial back the ketoanalogs and replace with EAAs until you are back in range with your calcium intake. Should serum calcium go too high with this approach, even though vitamin D and vitamin K2 intake is optimal, EAAs are your best bet. At this point, it's probably good to consult a medical professional to balance BUN and serum calcium.

Now keep in mind, this is a replacement for food, so the amounts needed may feel quite high and taking the required number of tablets can be quite cumbersome if you can't find a powdered form.

Bioavailable protein

If you are restricting protein and replacing the difference with essential amino acids in any form, it is also important you make the protein, and therefore nitrogen that you are consuming, count as much as possible. You can do this by consuming the most bioavailable forms of protein, as measured by their DIAAS (digestible indispensable amino acid) score, as seen on page 65 (Figure 6). As a general rule, animal proteins are more bioavailable than plant proteins and ruminants are better than poultry. For example, choosing grass-fed beef over protein from peas will just about double the usable amino acids from that protein for you, while keeping nitrogen intake the same. I know this won't make many vegan advocates happy, but in the case of high BUN, plant proteins are giving you a higher burden of nitrogen for every gram of usable amino acids.

The good news for vegetarians out there: there is hope. Whey protein, eggs, goat-milk and sheep-milk-based products are even higher on the DIAAS score list than grass-fed beef. So these are excellent options if you want to make optimal use of your nitrogen with highly bioavailable protein sources and are not sensitive to eggs or dairy.

Chitosan

As mentioned in the supplement section (page 145), chitosan reduced BUN by up to 40% with 12 weeks of daily usage in one study.[1] Refer to the chitosan section for more information.

Uric acid

Uric acid is a very interesting compound. Actually, humans are among the very few animals that have evolved to lose their genetic ability to break it down effectively with the enzyme called uricase. Uric acid is a byproduct of your metabolism of purines, which are contained in many plant- and animal-based foods. However, contrary to popular belief, food is not our main source of purines, which we'll explore further in a bit. Interestingly, the animals that have retained their uricase enzyme also retained their ability to produce their own vitamin C, which humans and guinea pigs also cannot do. So, we genetically already have higher levels of uric acid than other mammals. This also predisposes us to metabolic syndrome, which then causes uric acid levels to rise even more. This begs the question why evolution selected for these particular traits. Some hypotheses include longevity through antioxidant effects, similar to vitamin C, better blood pressure control even when salt is scarce, and even making us smarter.

The important thing to understand is that, while low kidney function will slow down the excretion of uric acid in late stages, thereby increasing blood uric acid levels, in many cases what pathologically raises uric acid in the first place is not kidney disease. Metabolic syndrome, which is in turn induced by a diet high in oxidized seed oils and processed carbs, is the more likely culprit in the general population. If you are starting out with a high uric acid level and you have not been on the program for at least a month or two, don't despair just yet. It's very possible your uric acid levels will come down once your body has adapted to a healthier way of eating and you have increased your insulin sensitivity. Keep an eye on the trend and how it's developing, not just the absolute values. Compare your new test result with the old one and if it's going down, keep going even if you haven't reached the normal range just yet.

So how about reducing your purine intake from food? Purine levels are all over the place among plant- and animal-based foods. Beef, for example, is lower than soy, mung beans or white beans and on par with lentils. But the body doesn't process all purines equally. It's not that simple. It is true that meat contains purines that are more readily converted to uric acid and plant purines contribute less to the total uric acid pool, with dairy being the notable alternative that actually seems to lower the production of uric acid.

However, most of the uric acid we produce is in fact synthesized not from purines in the diet, but from the breakdown of our own DNA.[2] As a 2012 article from *Advances in Chronic Kidney Disease* put it: 'Dietary purines contribute a relatively minor fraction to urate [uric acid] synthesis in most people; therefore, their reduction affords only a modest opportunity for disease control. That possibility broadens with the understanding that much endogenous synthesis is driven by fructose.'[3]

All of that said, a 2022 cohort study examined the effect of uric acid-lowering therapy on kidney disease progression and found that lowering uric acid levels pharmaceutically can actually make it even worse. Taking uric-acid-lowering medications increased the risk of progressing to an eGFR below 60 ml/min if patients had only slightly elevated uric acid (up to 8 mg/dl) and made little difference in patients with uric acid higher than 8 mg/dl.[4]

Another study in cell culture recently examined the effects

of high uric acid levels on apoptosis (programmed cell death) and found that levels up to 10 mg/dl only marginally increased cell death compared to the normal range. At 20 mg/dl is where they saw almost a doubling in apoptosis rates.[5]

This further supports the notion that uric acid might well serve a protective role, and pharmaceutically lowering it might not be necessary or beneficial for slightly elevated levels. When levels creep into the 8-10 mg/dl range, lowering it with non-pharmaceutical interventions is likely to be a sensible approach. Keep in mind that endogenous production from DNA break-down and synthesis driven by fructose are far greater contributors to uric acid levels than intake of dietary purines.

If limiting dietary purines is indicated, replacing part of your protein intake with dairy, like raw grass-fed A2 cheeses or whey protein powder, can be a sensible option, since dairy seems to actually lower the risk of elevated uric acid levels. Of course, you have to take into account your personal biology, as dairy usually is not recommended. However, in this case, you might want to take the hit on your immune system, even if you're sensitive, to get the protective effects for uric acid levels.

The effect of dairy on uric acid levels is hypothesized to be due to specific peptides (part of the milk and whey proteins) downregulating uric acid synthesis and increasing excretion rates.[6] Dairy products contain relevant amounts of phosphorus so, if those levels are elevated, analyze your phosphorus intake overall and possibly consider a non-aluminum phosphate binder; this will come with its own risks of mostly gastrointestinal origin. For more on phosphate, refer to page 82.

If you have been on a seed-oil-free, mostly ketogenic, clean diet for months and you have even replaced part of your protein intake with dairy, but your uric acid level still hasn't come down enough, there might be another way to significantly decrease uric acid and even creatinine levels. An extract of *T. Bellerica* contains about 1% chebulic acid and has been shown in one study to be able to reduce creatinine[7] and therefore increase kidney function by a whopping 24% while reducing uric acid levels by 34% after about 24 weeks of usage. Dosing was set at 1000 mg of *T. Bellerica* twice per day. Commercial products are available in the US, and some other countries offer a similar product in 'Haritaki', although the exact content of chebulic acid might not be known.

You might also be able to decrease your levels of uric acid by supplementing with tart/sour cherry or quercetin. You might be fine with widely available forms of these supplements, or you might want to try something more advanced like alpha-glycosyl isoquercitin or liposomal preparations, which are more bioavailable than standard quercetin.

Electrolytes

If levels of any electrolytes are elevated and you are not consuming excessive amounts in supplement form (usual suspects are exogenous ketone powders, ketoanalogs and mineral supplements, but it's best to double check), it makes sense to work with your doctor. Your doctor can prescribe a potassium or non-aluminum phosphate binder, or work with you to adjust vitamin D or ketoanalog dosage if calcium levels are too high, or even restrict sodium if it's elevated.

Phosphate and potassium

In the later stages of PKD, we can often see build-up of phosphate and potassium because excretion is just not working optimally anymore. There is the option of getting phosphate binders prescribed by your doctor and this is probably a good idea when your levels are elevated. For potassium, there are also pharmaceutical binders on the market, if restricting dietary intake is not enough. You can lower potassium content of vegetables by soaking them in water before cooking or you can choose lower-potassium foods in general. Tables listing potassium content of different foods can be found online easily. It makes sense to discuss a realistic daily potassium target with your doctor and tailoring your intake to stay below it.

I have included a chart (Figure 7) giving phosphate levels of protein sources by their protein content, so you can choose protein sources that give you the most protein with the least amount of phosphate. Lower milligrams are better. You will need this only if your phosphate blood levels are elevated.

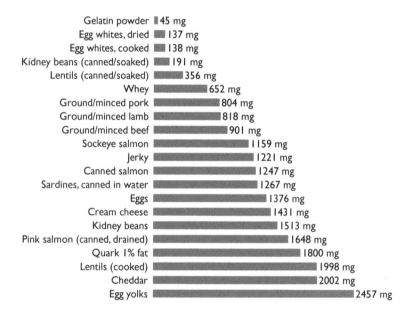

Figure 7: Phosphate to protein ratio showing phosphorus content of foods in milligrams per 100 grams of protein.

Hemoglobin

Hemoglobin is the iron-containing protein complex that is in our red blood cells and gives them their color. Hemoglobin levels

Reversing PKD

can decrease over time in PKD; this is called anemia. In fact, most people with late-stage kidney disease also develop anemia. There are basically two possible components to this condition, the most common in kidney disease being low production of EPO (erythropoietin), which stimulates the bone marrow to produce red blood cells. As kidney disease progresses, EPO production goes down and hemoglobin goes down with it. However, if EPO levels are okay, hemoglobin can also be affected by low bioavailable iron. Contrary to popular belief, this is usually not caused by low iron intake and also not remedied by iron supplementation or injections. Especially when you are eating adequate amounts of red meat, iron intake should be more than sufficient, even to the point of iron overload, especially in males and in females who are not menstruating. In this case, regular blood donations are critical to keep iron below toxic levels.

Please note, ferritin is not an accurate measure of iron status, even if this is a common assumption. Ferritin is an iron-carrying protein that's used inside the cell. The blood test that is usually employed to measure ferritin levels measures it outside the cell. This is usually a symptom of disease and inflammation because ferritin is not supposed to leak out. In theory, the best serum ferritin level would be zero, as all of it would be contained inside the cells, not the serum.

Now if your iron intake is good because you are eating adequate amounts of red meat, what could be another cause of low hemoglobin?

One very important dietary factor in the production of EPO is vitamin A in its natural form, retinol. Several studies show that supplementation with vitamin A increased blood levels of hemoglobin and stimulation of EPO production.[8] The synthesis of heme, which is at the center of hemoglobin, is also dependent on adequate copper levels.[9] It has long been known that copper deficiency can also lead to a deficiency in hemoglobin.

Since copper needs to be balanced with zinc, it makes

84

sense to find a combined product if you are considering supplementation. The optimal ratio seems to be about 1:15, so 15 mg of zinc for every mg of copper. There are several products on the market with this ratio.

For vitamin A, things get a little bit trickier. Most products on the market contain retinyl palmitate, which is a much cheaper synthetic form of retinol. Your best bet for finding real retinol is either a very clean straight fish liver oil supplement or one that contains an extract from fish liver. One brand out there still making a product like this is Bluebonnet. Their 10,000 IU vitamin A product is made from fish liver instead of synthetic vitamin A. This is an adequate daily dose.

Another great source for both copper and vitamin A is of course grass-fed beef or lamb liver. I am aware this is an acquired taste and I had to eat it about 10 times to finally be able to appreciate, or at least tolerate the taste. You can find a basic recipe later in this book (page 223).

So how do we integrate all this into a daily routine that is tasty, fun and sustainable? What's the schedule? Well, everyone will have to find their own way, but I can give you some insights into how I do it on a daily basis next and then an overview of the basic structure.

Chapter 7

Weekly schedule: timing

Example daily routine for ketogenic days

I usually start a standard ketogenic day waking up naturally without an alarm clock around 7:00 am. When I need to get up earlier than that, I will use an app called 'sleep cycle', which will wake me up during a 30-minute window before my desired wake-up time, when I am most awake. This prevents most of the groggy feeling going along with waking up to an alarm clock on most days.

Usually the first thing I do is drink ½ liter of hydrogen-rich water before I do anything else.

I will then proceed to sit in front of my NIR (near infrared) light bulbs for 15 minutes while reading a book. I will then use my Waterpik with some ozonated water, tongue scraping afterwards on some days, followed by a shower. I will usually listen to an interesting podcast while doing this. The shower is equipped with an activated charcoal filter. I use natural soap made with just coconut oil and goat's milk and for shampoo, if needed, I use ghassoul clay followed by an apple cider vinegar rinse. After the shower I might apply some natural oil- and baking soda-based deodorant and some homemade jojoba-based facial oil (see page 237).

I will then proceed to the kitchen, filling my glass-and-stainless-steel-only electric kettle with a litre of filtered water, setting it to a 90°C target temperature to make the optimal brew from my mold-free coffee beans in a double-walled French press with no plastic parts.

I will then make my bulletproof coffee: about 20 grams raw-milk grass-fed butter, 18 grams C8 MCT oil and sometimes 5-10 grams raw organic cocoa butter in the glass-and-steel blender, wait for three minutes until the coffee is done and then blend it up.

I will then take my fish oil and vitamin D with the first sip and proceed to the office. Depending on what the plan is for the day, I might either take a coffee in a normal glass, or in a contigo autoseal travel mug, equipped with a stainless steel shaker ball like body builders use, so I can shake up the hot coffee every now and then. Be cautious when choosing your travel mug, as the ones with the wrong mechanism can explode on you with this type of drink!

I will then slowly drink this coffee over an hour or so. Sometimes I will take a tablespoon of lecithin, some betaine HCl or pancreatin with it when I get the feeling my digestion might need a boost that morning. This is especially important for anyone who gets nauseous with lots of fat.

Come about 1:00 pm, it's lunchtime. If I'm on the go I will have something I prepared the day before, as I do not like to depend on restaurant food. It's usually worse than what I can make at home and it's expensive. If I haven't been able to prepare anything, I will usually combine stuff from the supermarket rather than going to a restaurant. This way I can read the ingredients and have a far greater selection. Lunch will usually consist of grass-fed meat and organic veggies topped with some saturated or monounsaturated fat. Whatever I eat, I will usually add a tablespoon of C8 MCT oil. I will add to that my mineral supplements which might contain a wide array of different minerals, adjusted to my personal hair-mineral analysis. At the very least my regimen will contain 500 mg of elemental magnesium, from either magnesium malate or citrate. This is also when I take most of my supplements for basic nutrition, such as vitamins, prebiotics and probiotics.

I might follow it up right after with dessert, such as home-made raw-milk *l. reuteri* yogurt with some monk fruit sweetener, 90% dark Lindt chocolate, raw organic macadamia nuts, homemade whey protein balls or grass-fed beef jerky. I might also have some raw-milk Parmigiano Reggiano cheese; however, you need to make sure you are neither sensitive to cheese or yogurt, nor have high phosphorus levels before adding either to your regimen. Lots of people react to casein (milk protein) and don't even know it because they never stop consuming it and therefore never experience how they feel without it.

Dinner is usually around 6-7:00 pm and will be very similar to what I had at lunch. I might stir some collagen powder into whatever sauce or dessert I'm having too, and might even have that with a shot of glycine and NAC dissolved in water. (I sometimes call this biohacker's lemonade, as it tastes pretty good.) Of course, C8 MCT oil will also be drizzled on this meal. This is also the time I'll have a small serving of berries on some days. They are best combined with a calcium source like the dairy we talked about before, bone broth or a simple clean calcium supplement to bind up any oxalates they contain.

Whatever time the sun goes down, I will put on my blue-blocking glasses and switch on some red LED lights when just lounging around on the couch, or a larger halogen light with a dimmer switch that also emits a nice warm natural light and doesn't disrupt my circadian rhythm too much. All screens I might be using are switched to night mode, so they emit much less blue light than during the daytime. If I watch something in the evening it will be something informative or funny most of the time so I give my body a chance to wind down. Crime shows or news reports are usually not a great idea in general, but much less if you want a good night's sleep. Get off the cortisol carousel!

After dinner I might have some autophagy tea (see page 234) or an apple cider vinegar nighttime drink.

I then brush my teeth with some organic calcium-hydroxapatite-containing toothpaste and use some unwaxed dental floss. I use a super-soft natural toothbrush to keep my enamel intact. This is also the time to take the rest of my cyst-growth-blocking supplements such as quercetin, ginkgo biloba, bioavailable curcumin and berberine, or, if I am on a toxin-adsorption day, chitosan, activated charcoal, modified citrus pectin, or possibly even cholestyramine if I am on an endotoxin or mold detox.

I might even use the time I'm asleep for some more healing measures by putting some essential oils in the diffuser next to the bed. Some of my favorites are pine needle scotch for immune system function,[1] cinnamon for mitigating endotoxin-induced damage[2] or sweet orange to nourish beneficial bacteria and strengthen the gut lining.[3]

The PKDproof program weekly schedule

Now that you've seen how a standard day might look for me, let's go into detail on what is important in designing your regular weekly schedule on the PKDproof program.

Keto days

About five to six days per week should be keto days, fewer if you are a child, pregnant or breast-feeding. More keto days equals less cyst growth but a higher risk for side effects of chronic ketosis that we talked about before (page 13).

On those days, as described in my personal schedule, start with a bulletproof coffee, follow up with a lunch of mostly meat and

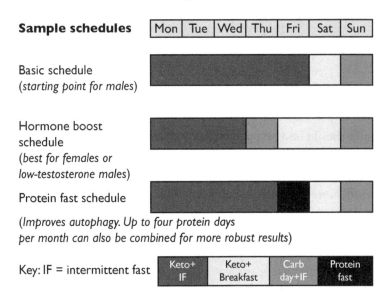

Figure 8: Weekly sample schedules showing carb, keto and protein fast days. (You can mix and match for individualized goals)

vegetables drizzled in fat around 1:00 pm, and finish with dinner around 7:00-8:00 pm containing similar foods. If you're going to have a small serving of good fruit, dinner is the time to have it.

Carb days

One or two days per week should therefore be carb days (page 217). On those days you can have a liberal quantity of good starches. If you are going to binge on something in the medium or even bad category of foods (page 39), this is probably the day to do it; however, these are not 'cheat days'. If you start treating them like they are, you will quickly find yourself in a world of trouble, potentially always thinking about the next 'hit'. Been there, done that. Rather, keep your 'cheating' to occasions that you have no control over, such as events you've been invited to.

On those days, make sure to have charcoal handy and take it with sub-par foods.

Protein-fasting days

One day a week, or even three to four days a month back-to-back, should be a protein fasting day. On these days we reap even higher autophagy benefits because we keep mTOR (page 12) to the absolute minimum by minimizing protein intake. Raise your protein intake on the rest of the days of the week accordingly so you hit the daily average calculated (page 66).

The advantage of a protein fast compared to a traditional full water fast is that you keep things moving in your gut, which means whenever your body unavoidably dissolves fat cells, the toxins that are stored inside can be excreted through your gut. In a pure water fast, these toxins get reabsorbed and redistributed throughout the body, which can leave them stored in a worse place than they came from – worst-case even in the brain, which can lead to new health issues like Alzheimer's disease or Parkinson's down the road. More on this in the Protein fasting section on page 131.

Now, as your blood glucose levels will be dropping below their usual levels, this is the day to incorporate some modest glutamine inhibition to starve PKD cells even more. Refer to Chapter 11 on glutamine-blockers for a list of options and strategies (see page 152). These interventions are more effective the lower your blood glucose is, so you might want to consider multiple protein-fasting days back-to-back once a month instead of a weekly regimen.

Adjustments

If some of your laboratory parameters are out of range, check back with Chapter 6 Adjustments for low kidney function, to see if you need to make any changes to the Bulletproof Diet template described in Chapter 4.

Vegetarian and vegan diets

There is a lot of fear-mongering going on, especially in the kidney health community, regarding animal proteins. If you're coming from an ethical perspective, I recommend you research how many smaller animals are getting killed in mass farming of crops, and how much natural habitat is getting destroyed to make room for these fields. Rabbits, deer, frogs, birds… millions of these animals are getting killed in industrial-scale farming every year. A good starting point is the Steven L. Davis study that found eating large herbivores like beef might actually result in fewer deaths worldwide than if all humans were consuming a vegan diet.[4] The study has been criticized for underestimating the number of deaths resulting from crop production, so the data can be interpreted to even more strongly suggest a large herbivore-based diet.[5]

When you stick to grass-fed beef there is no habitat destruction, no killing of small animals and about 300 to 400 kg of highly nutritious meat for every one cow that is slaughtered. If you're considering going without meat from a kidney health perspective, keep reading.

If you have a kidney health problem, should you be vegetarian? Or even vegan? What are the arguments for and against this lifestyle from a kidney health perspective? How do proponents of vegetarian and vegan diets justify recommending these diets for PKD? The reasons are often vague and given in broad brushstrokes: 'alkalinity', 'lowering blood pressure', 'lowering blood sugar', 'lowering cholesterol', 'improving antioxidant levels' and so on. Some of these goals are either easily reached and even surpassed with our approach in this book, like optimal urine pH, lowering blood pressure and lowering blood sugar, while others are not worth attaining at all, like lowering cholesterol. Cholesterol is not an issue. High cholesterol is a result of either ongoing inflammation from a bad diet or a normal physiological response to a ketogenic diet. Some of their claims also don't even mean anything, like improving antioxidant levels. More on that later. And most proponents aren't even addressing the downsides of a vegan diet.

There is still a presupposition in many patients' minds that somehow protein is bad, animal protein being even worse, and red meat being the worst of the worst. But what does 'bad' actually mean in this context? Whatever it means to you, the fact is that your kidneys need high-quality proteins in adequate amounts to retain and restore proper function. This means a high DIAAS score is essential (see page 65), especially if you want to consume less total protein and fewer toxins from pesticides and plant-based antinutrients. For more on red meat, refer to page 102.

If being vegetarian still is your preference, whey protein, soft-boiled eggs and goat- as well as sheep-milk-based products have the most bioavailable vegetarian protein. (But you need to make sure you're not casein sensitive first.)

High DIAAS score options are quite limited for vegans though, as most of them are laden with antinutrients. The cleanest one seems to be hemp-based protein, but the DIAAS score for this is not looking great. So you will need to find organic vegan protein powder blends that are low in pesticides and mimic the amino acid composition of animal protein sources, giving you a high DIAAS score, but leaving you with the antinutrient burden.

Sorry, vegans!

The lightning-bolt pattern: An illusion of improved function

'But eGFR improved when x person went vegan!' – I'm glad we get the chance to clear up this critical misconception. As we discussed before (page 63), eGFR (estimated glomerular filtration rate) is an estimate, based on creatinine levels. All things being equal, this estimation is fairly accurate, but it makes one central assumption: most people's muscle mass is in a certain standard range. Muscle constantly releases creatinine into the blood, which is then filtered out by the kidneys.

This is why, for example, body builders tend to get lower eGFR readings. Their muscle mass is higher than that of the reference population, producing more creatinine that needs to be filtered. Even if they have the same function as the next person, their calculated eGFR is going to be lower, as they start with a higher creatinine level to begin with.

When people go vegan, the vast majority inadvertently reduce their protein intake, and even if they try to match it, plant proteins are less bioavailable and less effective at producing muscle, so in most cases people lose muscle mass when they switch to a vegan diet. This gives them a lower level of creatinine production, which then looks like function has improved according to eGFR. In reality, they have just lost muscle mass and function has stayed the same. In the following years, we can usually see them continuing on the same slope of decline, leading to the 'lightning bolt pattern' (see Figure 9) when they graph their creatinine and eGFR test results.

We see a continuing decline in eGFR and then what looks like an almost instantaneous 'improvement' when they go vegan, followed by the same continuing rate of decline. No improvement in function has been achieved, but this common misinterpretation usually costs patients crucial years to preserve and increase function, which depends on proper protein bioavailability. Only if muscle mass stays the same or increases can improvements in creatinine be taken as actual function improvement.

Muscle mass is one of the most important factors for a long, healthy life, so embarking on any strategy that reduces it might be one of the most foolish things you could do.[6]

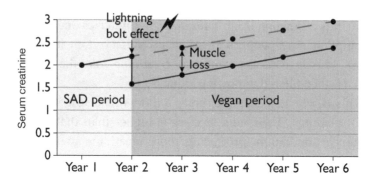

Figure 9: The lightning-bolt effect – Switching from a standard American diet (SAD) to a vegan diet in PKD results in initial decreased serum creatinine, which does not mirror an increase in kidney function, but an inadvertent decreased protein intake

An alternative to measuring eGFR using creatinine is estimating function based on cystatin-c, which is much more consistent. However, it is not possible to compare eGFR based on creatinine to eGFR based on cystatin-c directly.

One study from the 80s actually analyzed changes in creatinine in people on a low-protein diet, and, as if it wasn't obvious enough, they found this exact pattern. To quote from the study: 'Muscle mass and plasma creatinine fell simultaneously in several patients. [...] A fall in plasma creatinine may not be due to improved GFR but instead to altered creatinine metabolism.' [7] In plain English, this means patients had a different creatinine metabolism as a result of their lower muscle mass. Figure 10 is an image from the study showing the different participants' results.

Figure 10 (opposite): The correlation between muscle mass and creatinine metabolism in three patients representing different types of response, based on data in the study by Lucas et al[7]

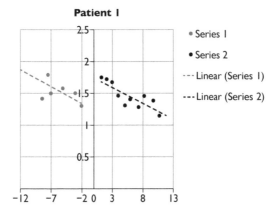

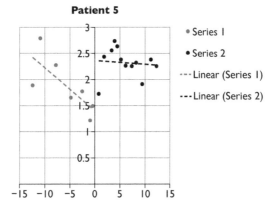

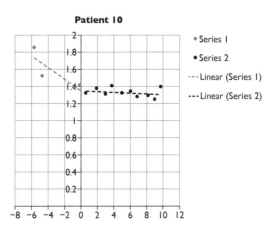

What to eat on the road

Whenever you do encounter a 'cheat day', be it at a friend's wedding, a birthday or whatever else life might throw at you, don't despair. Just have some activated charcoal on hand to mitigate whatever sub-par foods you might have consumed that day.

Pro tip: If you suspect you might have eaten bad fats that are high in linoleic acid, like sunflower oil or canola oil, it makes sense to consume a lot of saturated fat right afterwards so your body has a chance to choose better fats over those high omega-6 oils you might have just consumed. A convenient method of quickly consuming saturated fat to offset vegetable oils could be to eat some butter, coconut oil, high-fat cheese, an avocado, or 85%+ dark chocolate, etc.

If you ever opt to eat grains 'on the road', which I highly recommend against, some science suggests that an extract from a special type of seaweed called bladderwrack actually binds gluten in the gut.[8] So if you are planning on having that conventional pizza at your friend's birthday party once a year, bring your charcoal and bladderwrack capsules to prevent the worst from happening.

It's always a great idea to bring your own condiments when traveling. A small bottle of MCT oil, a portable saltshaker with great quality salt inside and a couple of small packets of grass-fed butter can go a long way to making many meals more conducive to a state of ketosis when you're traveling. Of course, it makes sense to schedule your carbohydrate refeed day for one of those days when you're on the road, to make things easier.

Among my favorite foods to eat at restaurants are:
* Poké bowls
* Avocado or cucumber sushi with MCT oil and salt (carb

day)
- Grass-fed steak and vegetables (check for seed oils)
- Gluten-free pizza (as a treat on a carb day, take charcoal)
- Salads with olive oil and vinegar, skip the dressing (check for seed oils)
- Grilled lamb and vegetables at Greek restaurants (check for seed oils).

Food ideas to take with you for eating on the road without kitchen access include:
- Homemade grass-fed beef meatballs
- Peeled carrots
- Dark chocolate
- Beef jerky
- Boiled eggs (soft is best)
- Macadamia nuts
- Jars of homemade panna cotta (refrigerate)
- Jars of homemade yogurt with berries, coconut shreds and nuts
- Parmigiano Reggiano or other raw-milk, grass-fed A2* cheese, if tolerated
- Grass-fed beef sausages
- Organic fruit (carb days)
- Homemade salad, extra vinaigrette dressing
- Homemade whey protein balls.

*Note: A2 casein is a more similar casein to human breast milk. It's found in the milk of sheep, goats and some select cow breeds.

Chapter 8

Common myths

Salt

The advice to limit salt consumption regardless of laboratory measurements is an outdated concept. A ketogenic diet requires up to four times the amount of salt compared to a high-carbohydrate diet as it becomes harder for the body to hold on to sodium. If you are currently on a salt-restricted diet, you can take your baseline blood pressure and then switch to the Bulletproof Diet for about a week. If your blood pressure rises by more than 5 mm Hg systolic or 3 mm Hg diastolic when you switch to a higher-salt diet, you are considered to be salt-sensitive according to medical professionals. This might indicate that you are potassium deficient, but since we are increasing potassium intake quite substantially when following this diet, it is very possible that your blood pressure will slowly improve over time.

Apart from blood pressure issues in salt-sensitive people who haven't addressed a likely potassium deficiency, there is nothing to be gained from doing anything but salting to taste. The body needs salt to stay hydrated. The more water you drink, the more salt you will need to keep the proper electrolyte balance. Your body will tell you what the proper balance is, if you listen to your taste buds. Of course, avoiding hidden salt in processed foods will also go a long way to making sure your body is actually taking in as much salt as it needs, but not too much.

Coffee

Similar to salt, coffee has been vilified in the kidney health and PKD communities. Doctors used to recommend against coffee for PKD patients in the past because of concerns that it might raise blood pressure or cause dehydration. However, more recent studies have shown that coffee may not be as harmful as previously thought. In fact, one cohort study from 2018 actually showed that coffee drinkers had slightly smaller kidneys and better kidney function, even though the difference was not statistically significant.[1]

Considering most of these people probably consumed coffee that was contaminated with mold toxins[2] and did not drink it in the context of nutritional ketosis, as we are doing, this gives even more weight to the mechanisms in coffee that actually seem to benefit PKD, like the increase in ketones and autophagy, the mTOR inhibition that caffeine produces, and of course the antioxidants fighting inflammation, which is chronically elevated in PKD. So go ahead, brew yourself that nice high-fat cup of mold-free coffee.

In addition, coffee has actually been shown to reduce uric acid by inhibiting synthesis from purines and increasing excretion through urine. Decaf works, too, but caffeinated works better.

So drink up![3]

Red meat

Red meat too has been unrightfully vilified for decades now and it might be beyond the scope of this book to convince some of the old guard that are still afraid of this basic food group. Most of the bad press that red meat has received can be traced back to a number of epidemiological studies that lumped together all types of red meat, not differentiating between meats of different quality, such as grass-fed, organic or conventional, or even processed versus unprocessed meats. In addition, because of the so-called 'unhealthy user bias', the people who eat the most red meat are also the people who are least likely to follow other public health recommendations, such as not smoking or drinking and exercising regularly. This leads to confounding factors in the research that can never be controlled for entirely. Additionally, look at countries where eating red meat is considered healthy, such as parts of Asia. A pooled prospective cohort study of eight Asian countries found that 'Red meat intake was inversely associated with CVD (cardiovascular disease) mortality in men and with cancer mortality in women in Asian countries', meaning higher red meat intake was associated with lower disease risk in these cases.[4]

In these countries, the unhealthy user bias still exists, but it does not bias the results against red meat, and so the correlation that led to the vilification of red meat, disappears.

So now that we are clear on the fact that red meat probably doesn't increase your risk of CVD or cancer, let's recap the benefits. As we discussed before, the ruminants that make our red meat have one big advantage over those animals that have white meat, such as pigs or chicken – they have multiple stomachs, which gives them the unique ability to convert polyunsaturated omega-6 fats, such as linoleic acid, which we want to avoid almost at all costs (see page 47), to healthy saturated fat. This is why the fat in red meat is so uniquely beneficial. It is very low in polyunsaturated fatty acids. If your beef is grass-fed and grass-finished, you're getting even more benefits because of its higher and more diverse nutrient content.

Additionally, as it is vital to consume adequate amounts of protein to repair and maintain kidney tissue, you will quickly find that a diet without meat makes it very difficult to reach your daily protein target, especially if you want to steer clear of highly processed protein powders.

Chapter 9

Lifestyle strategies

Sauna and infrared light therapy

Sauna and infrared light have a myriad of benefits, especially when combined. As we discussed, the PKD mutations primarily mess with the structure of certain proteins. If you have a PKD1 mutation, it's the PC-1 protein, and if it's PKD2, then it's the PC-2 protein. These proteins are so-called membrane proteins – specifically, they are part of tiny hair-like structures on the cell membranes called cilia.

Now, you might carry the mutation, but this does not mean that you don't have healthy cells that express the original, not the mutated, version of these genes. Most people, who have the heterozygous mutation have one healthy copy and one mutated copy of the gene. So, to make up for those damaged proteins that are built by the mutated version of the gene, it becomes all the more important we make sure that the proteins built by the healthy version of the gene actually are built, or folded, correctly.[1]

That is to say, when part of your PC-1 is already damaged because of the mutation, it's vital to make sure the rest gets folded correctly. Believe it or not, about 30% of proteins are misfolded right off the bat, in anybody.[2] Not just in PKD. So, there's room for improvement!

Now, there is something that can actually help improve protein-folding: heat shock proteins (HSPs). These are your body's little helpers when it comes to making sure proteins fold the way they're supposed to. Saunas are a fantastic way to ramp up your body's production of HSPs. By doing so, you're aiding your system in getting those proteins to fold correctly, which is super-helpful when you're dealing with PKD and already have those damaged PC-1 or PC-2 proteins. Now, additionally you are also excreting toxins through sweat in the sauna, which can help your body even to get rid of toxins that would normally leach from your fat tissue for the rest of your life. Needless to say, this takes a further burden off the kidneys.

Beyond saunas, red light therapy can provide additional benefits. It has long been known that red and infrared light increases mitochondrial efficiency. Animal models show that red light can improve respiration and even rescue cells after hypoxia.[3] As you know, PKD patients are dealing with the Warburg effect – that is, impaired mitochondrial respiration and energy production without the use of oxygen. Red light therapy's beneficial effect on mitochondrial respiration could potentially push cells away from relying on fermentation and back towards healthy aerobic metabolism in the mitochondria (see page 6). Specifically, it does this by 'knocking off' bound nitric oxide (NO) from an important mitochondrial enzyme called cytochrome c oxidase (CCO). When CCO absorbs the red light, it changes its shape to free the bound-up NO, which then makes it able to restart its processing of oxygen, effectively increasing oxygen uptake (respiration) in the mitochondria, which then means the PC-1 protein will sense more oxygen and tell PC-2 to let more calcium into the cell. This could in theory help prevent new cyst growth as that is largely a result of chronic low respiration.

This mechanism was originally discovered in cancer studies.[4] Out of an abundance of caution I personally recommend sticking to classic-style near-infrared heat bulbs, since they provide a broad spectrum of light which is more similar to the sun. Now ranges of light frequencies, such as those emitted from LEDs, haven't been tested for nearly as long, so I will only use those when traveling. There has been some research suggesting a potential negative effect from pure visible red light LEDs in PKD, which is why I always use a combination of near-infrared and red LEDs at the very least; however, my favorite are near-infrared bulbs, like the ones grandma used for all sorts of ailments. They give you a balanced range of frequencies similar to the sun. Of all the frequencies, the ones in the visible red and near-infrared range penetrate the deepest into biological tissues. Far-infrared does not penetrate as deeply into the skin, so it's unlikely to have direct benefits for the kidney.

The best of both worlds is to find an infrared sauna that uses heat bulbs and emits very little EMF. If the wiring in your sauna irradiates you with electromagnetic waves while you are trying to relax, your body will be in fight or flight mode and detox is going to shut off for the most part. The easiest thing to do is to get a trifield meter or similar and test whatever sauna you are considering for magnetic fields. You can add your own infrared bulbs if necessary, and you can even position them outside to shine in through the glass. There are shielded near-infrared saunas on the market that use incandescent near-infrared bulbs as their heat source. It goes without saying that phones, smart watches, etc. must be in airplane mode and wi-fi routers need to be switched off as well if you want detox to work.

Optimizing sleep

Sleep is paramount for all types of healing; our grandmas knew this. And PKD is no exception. Melatonin, the sleep hormone, has actually been shown to reduce cyst growth in a fly model of PKD[5] and reduce blood pressure in humans.[6] In any case, it is a potent antioxidant that has huge benefits. While I totally understand why people opt for supplementation with melatonin, which can be very helpful, especially as production drops with age, I like to begin by optimizing the environment for producing melatonin ourselves.

Melatonin production usually begins about two hours after the last ray of blue light has hit your retina. For most people today, this is when they close their eyes in bed. You might be tired enough by that point that you can still fall asleep, albeit this sleep will be far less restorative than if you had skipped the blue light a couple of hours before bed. High adenosine levels in the brain that have built up during the day make this happen, but without adequate levels of melatonin you will be falling asleep much later than if you had skipped the blue light for a couple of hours before bed. This hormonal state resembles passing out from exhaustion in the middle of the day much more than it does a traditional good night's sleep, and will be far less restorative and healing.

A healthy circadian rhythm is what helps you get more restorative and peaceful sleep as your melatonin levels naturally rise in the evening. This is very important since melatonin is a critical hormone to induce autophagy during the night. Your body gets its clues for increasing melatonin levels from sensing light in your environment, mainly the absence of blue light. Now as you probably remember from physics class, white light contains blue light, too. Modern light sources such as fluorescent lights and LEDs contain an even higher amount of blue light than traditional light sources such as incandescent and halogen. Luckily, halogen lights are still available widely and if you reduce their intensity with a dimmer switch, they shift much more towards the red spectrum. Our bodies interpret this as evening, similar to a fireplace or a bonfire in early human evolution. There are apps for the computer and your smart phone to greatly reduce the blue light output, but the best approach is just to use dark orange or deep red glasses about two hours before bedtime. For a cheap option, look for green laser protection glasses. They're red, because they block out green light (and blue light, for that matter). They might look dorky, but they work! You will notice feeling a lot more at peace in the evenings as your melatonin levels naturally rise. Add some chamomile tea and skip the news stories and crime shows for even better results.

There is also the option of supplementing melatonin, as mentioned. Just note that most products contain way more than your body will ever produce and therefore tend to lead to dependency. It's possible that high doses of melatonin supplementation might help in reducing PKD cyst growth in humans, as it has been shown to do in flies[5] but if you ever run out or forget to take it, you might be in for a couple of rough nights. So choose wisely. The best form to take is as a sublingual spray, which has much better absorption than tablets or capsules. Dosage: 0.5 mg, increase as needed.

By this point you are already well informed on the basics of reversing PKD. Now you might be wondering how you will know if you are on the right track. Well, we will cover that next, and also give you the tools necessary to avoid being blindsided by your next lab test.

Chapter 10

Tracking your progress

Tracking your progress at home

What to measure and how to interpret it

Whenever you are embarking on a new lifestyle strategy, it is important to make sure that it is actually working for you. To ensure this, there are several tests that you can do at home regularly, in addition to your regular blood testing at the nephrologist's office. We'll take a look at how to interpret these tests, as well as some of the basics for interpreting lab tests done at the doctor's office. This will not be a comprehensive manual on how to interpret blood results as this would probably take a whole other book, but I will go into some of the markers that can help you tailor your diet to your personal needs.

pH

The first thing that your cells need in order to be able to repair themselves is actually a great milieu. You can think of your body's pH as being somewhat similar to the thermostat in a room. A lower than optimal pH represents a room that's too cold while a higher than optimal pH represents a room that is too hot. In both cases, anyone in the room won't be able to perform optimally

– just as cellular functions are impaired by a suboptimal pH milieu. Many people in the health world keep touting a so-called 'alkaline diet'. While it is true that most people nowadays tend to be more on the acidic end of the spectrum, you can, most definitely, be too alkaline as well.

While it is true that your blood's pH is tightly regulated and will only get out of range in very serious health conditions, the body uses different mechanisms to keep a stable pH, including buffering systems that neutralize excess acids or bases. The kidneys are part of this system, excreting the byproducts of these processes. This is why urine pH can give us clues as to how actively the body is working to maintain its pH balance. This is why we should strive to be in the optimal urine pH range, which is between 6.5 and 7.

Measuring second morning urine means you get up in the morning, pee, drink pure water and skip any meds, supplements or food for the time being. Wait until you have to pee again and then use that to measure your urine pH. You can use pH strips, which don't have to be calibrated as such; however, they can be a little inaccurate, which is why I like digital pH meters. Get one that is a little higher in quality, preferably one with a round top, not a rectangular one. The round ones tend to be higher quality.

You need to recalibrate these every so often. You can keep the calibration solution in a jar somewhere on hand so you can quickly recalibrate and check the accuracy with no hassle. The solutions around pH 4-7 usually have a shelf-life of 6-12 months.

If your pH is below 6.5, you are most likely not eating enough non-starchy vegetables. Each of your two to three meals every day should be mostly non-starchy vegetables from the 'good' category (see page 39) by volume. This ensures a high intake of alkalizing minerals. You should also be taking 500-1000 mg of magnesium, beginning with the malate form, which also fuels your citric acid cycle, and if that's not alkalizing enough, proceeding to the citrate form, which will yield an even higher alkalizing effect.

If that is not enough to get you into the optimal urine pH zone, you probably need to add some sodium bicarbonate. Be aware, though, that this will neutralize your stomach acid, so it should preferably come in an enteric coated tablet or capsule so as to not impair your digestion too much. With or without coating, it is probably still best to take it away from food, optimally two hours after your evening meal, evening being the best time because, from a circadian rhythm perspective, your body wants to be more acidic in the morning and more alkaline at night. Alkalinity calms while acidity excites.

Blood pressure

First, let's define high blood pressure. Up until not too long ago, high blood pressure was diagnosed by doing three consecutive measurements at rest. Only if all of them were above 140:90 mm Hg was the patient considered to experience hypertension. Guidelines have been updated numerous times, and in 2017 the limit was lowered to 130:80. Needless to say, this resulted in a nice increase in profits for anyone in the business of selling blood pressure medication. The rationale for lowering this limit was not entirely convincing.

It's worth noting that a reading of 120:80 mm Hg is often considered ideal. Some doctors aim to correct blood pressure to levels lower than this, but achieving such low levels can be challenging without medication and may be artificially low for some people based on their fitness level and body type. Targeting such a low blood pressure level can also be a concern in itself as it can lead to fatigue and lethargy. Given these considerations and the potential side effects of blood pressure medications, you need to decide what your target blood pressure level will be, and if potentially correcting it below your biologically optimal level is worth it to you.

Now, in PKD it does make sense to keep blood pressure in the normal range because high pressure can actually damage the kidneys directly, and, as we know, any injury to the kidneys can also trigger cyst growth in that area.

While many PKD patients struggle with blood pressure problems, not everyone experiences this issue. This fact alone tells us that there is more to blood pressure issues than just being diagnosed with PKD. So naturally, it would make sense to look at all the interventions that can improve blood pressure in general and see how far those will take us.

Elevated blood pressure that does not stem from kidney disease or any other type of underlying condition is called primary hypertension and it is the most common type. In many, or arguably most, cases this is caused by insulin resistance (the condition in which the cells stop responding to normal levels of insulin; the pancreas is then triggered to produce more and more insulin to counteract this resistance). Luckily enough, the approaches outlined in this book will go a long way to addressing this root cause.

In addition to fixing insulin resistance by skipping processed carbs and seed oils and spending most, but not all, of your time in a ketogenic state, there are some other things you need to get right in order to optimize your cardiovascular system and thereby also blood pressure. You will find those in the section on supplements (page 173).

Ketones

Of course, in order to track your progress on the PKDproof Program it is a great idea to make sure that your body is actually producing ketones. Contrary to popular belief, it's not enough to use urine test strips or breath meters. They are simply not accurate. Ketones are critical to get PKD cells back to metabolizing oxygen and therefore stop their unlimited proliferation; the only method that makes sense is to test blood ketone levels at home regularly to make sure the diet is actually getting us closer to the goal.

The one and only way to do it is with a finger-prick blood meter, just like the ones diabetics use at home to gauge their blood glucose status. You can get ketone as well as glucose test strips for these and they work really well. You are looking for anything above 0.3 mmol/l, which is where nutritional ketosis officially starts. After your bulletproof coffee in the morning, you might already be higher than that.

Individual reactions to foods can be very different, and if you have a sub-clinical food sensitivity, even ketogenic foods can actually raise blood sugar due to a cortisol spike. So, regularly testing ketone levels in the morning and one to two hours after meals is a great way to make sure you aren't eating anything that is compromising your success.

In the beginning, ketone levels might be a lot higher since your cells will still be struggling to use this new kind of fuel. As your body begins to adapt to a ketogenic diet like this, ketone levels are gradually going to come down. This is not a bad thing since it means your body is actually using ketones for energy and is efficiently producing just as much as it needs. The more adapted you become, the smaller the buffer that's needed in your blood, which is what we are actually measuring. Dr Cate Shanahan coined the term 'ketone flux' for this. You don't need or want a consistently high blood sugar level, and with ketones it is quite similar. It is not necessarily normal to have consistently high levels and can probably only be achieved through extreme fasting or ketone supplementation in the long term.

Levels are very individual as well, but anything over 0.3 mmol/l is considered nutritional ketosis.

There are no data for now that can say what level of ketones is required for cyst shrinkage. An early small study in humans did show a correlation between higher blood ketone levels and improvement in kidney function,[1] with the highest levels being around 3.0 mmol/l. However, many participants were new to a ketogenic diet so their bodies were not yet fully adapted. This would mean there was probably not a high level of ketone flux. You could also say their ketone buffers might have been more filled up than in a keto-adapted person as their cells were only beginning to learn how to use ketones for energy efficiently.

All we can say is that in the beginning phase, higher levels of ketones correlate with a higher improvement in kidney function. We do not know if in later stages high levels like this are still required or if ketone flux applies to PKD cells, too. That said, we should always strive to keep ketone levels as high as possible with a good diet, except for carb days where we rely on MCT oil to give us some background level of ketones. Keep a close eye on results and whenever you see levels dropping, look into the cause and adjust.

When you are able to predict the results after a couple of weeks of adjusting your diet, it's probably okay to switch to a more relaxed testing regimen. For example, you can re-test every couple of weeks just to make sure that your predictions are still accurate.

My personal experience was that the approach described in this book was sufficient to decrease kidney volume and increase GFR (glomerular filtration rate) by over 50 points over several years.

My personal ketone level began at 1-2 mmol/l on average and has gradually come down to 0.5-1.0 mmol/l after close to a decade in nutritional ketosis on most days.

Blood glucose

While you're at it, you might as well track your blood glucose (blood sugar) level, too. Especially fasting blood glucose can be interesting since it is elevated in many patients but should go down quickly with a proper diet. However, in some people who don't include carbohydrate refeeds, for example, fasting blood glucose can creep up over time, showing a chronic glucose deficiency that is getting offset by the body making new glucose out of muscle, a process called gluconeogenesis. This leads to diminishing returns on the ketogenic diet because of the chronically elevated blood glucose level even though carb intake remains minimal. When you see an elevated blood glucose reading in the morning, think stress or missing carb days and start to look for the cause.

Diet tracking

As we have discussed already, especially in the beginning it can be a great idea to track what you are actually eating so you can be sure that you really are achieving what you set out to do. My favorite app for this is called 'Cronometer' and it is a free app that anyone can use. You set the app as follows:

- Tracking carbohydrates as: Net carbs without sugar alcohols
- Set macro targets using: Ketogenic Calculator
- Select your keto program: Custom
- Grams of protein per kg of lean body mass: 1.4
- Grams of non-fiber carbohydrates per day: 40
- No athletic bonus.

Be sure to enter the most generic versions of the foods that you consume, since those will be pulled from the NCCDB, which has all the micronutrient, in addition to macronutrient, data available.

Pro tip: If you want to share details from the app with someone, just log in on your computer, navigate to the day in question and use the print function to print the page as a PDF that you can then share via email or messenger.

Tracking your progress with a provider

Laboratory results

Of course, you should use blood testing to your advantage and learn the basics of interpreting your results at home. Some of these can give insights into how to customize your diet based on your specific body and kidney function.

EGFR (estimated glomerular filtration rate)

Commonly misread as a percentage, the EGFR is calculated from your blood creatinine level and your age, as well as race and gender. It's the easiest way to quickly assess where you stand on your kidney function. This number is often categorized into stages of kidney dysfunction:

- \>90   ml/min: Stage 1
- 60-89   ml/min: Stage 2
- 45-59   ml/min: Stage 3A
- 30-44   ml/min: Stage 3B
- 15-29   ml/min: Stage 4
- <15   ml/min: Stage 5

However, stage 1 shouldn't even be called a stage, as function is completely normal and the sky is the limit here. My most recent lab test showed a cool 134 ml/min, my highest result yet. This number is not a percentage and it does not top out at 100, which is a common misconception.

Vitamins D and K2

Vitamin D is vital for immune system function and it's right in there with your natural killer cells fighting off viruses and bacterial infections, so you should always make sure to have a good blood level of vitamin D. The test we are looking for here is called 25-OH-D and you want the result to be somewhere between 60 and 90 ng/ml.

There are some convincing data to show that some famous respiratory viruses could basically have a 0% death rate (they kill nobody) whenever blood levels exceed 50 ng/ml.[2]

A good starting point for dosing, according to the Vitamin D Council, is 1000 IU vitamin D for every 25 lb (roughly 11 kg) of body weight per day. For example, a 150-pound man or woman would be taking 6000 IU per day. Your results may vary based on absorption and product quality, so it is paramount to test. Three to four weeks after beginning the supplementation is a good point in time to do it.

Now, vitamin D also has the function of shuttling calcium around your body. You can think of it as the truck carrying the load of calcium. However, it needs vitamin K2 to find its way; think of vitamin K2 as the truck driver. Without vitamin K2, an increased level of vitamin D will begin redistributing calcium deposits basically randomly throughout the body and it might end up in arteries or joints where we don't want it. So, an adequate level of vitamin K2 intake is paramount. This way, calcium will be liberated from arteries and joints and will be deposited where we need it: in bone and teeth.

Recommended intake for vitamin K2 is 200 mcg of the MK-7 form per day.

You can even find liquid supplements that incorporate both of these in the proper ratio.

Parathyroid hormone

This one is intricately linked with vitamin D intake. If your parathyroid hormone is too high, chances are that your vitamin D level is too low. In this case, start by taking the recommended amount of vitamin D daily. If PTH doesn't come down enough, get a 25-OH-D blood test to assess vitamin D status. Increase your dosage until you reach up to 90 ng/dl if necessary to get your PTH back in range.

Uric acid

As we discussed before, uric acid is a metabolite from the breakdown of purines, which occur in both animal and plant foods as well as our own DNA (page 6). It is excreted through the kidneys so it doesn't build up in the bloodstream. However, when kidney function is declining, blood levels of uric acid can go up as excretion gets impaired.

There is more on how to mitigate this in Chapter 6 on adjustments for low kidney function (see page 79).

BUN

Blood urea nitrogen, or sometimes just 'urea', is a waste product of protein metabolism. Protein is made up of individual amino acids that can then be reassembled into new proteins that act like little machines inside of our bodies.

Whenever amino acids from protein that we eat undergo a process called 'deamination', which is the removal of nitrogen from the amino acids by an enzyme, there is an excess of nitrogen that our kidneys need to get rid of. This is usually not a problem, but in later stages of kidney disease, there can be a build-up of nitrogen which is expressed in an elevated level of BUN on a blood test. Whenever you see an elevated level of BUN on your results, you might want to consider restructuring your protein intake.

There is more on this in Chapter 6: Adjustments for low kidney function (see page 73).

Cholesterol

The long-outdated science on cholesterol that most medical

professionals have learned in their careers is of no help to the patient with the goal of optimal health. It should be noted that standard cholesterol measurements do in no way, shape or form predict heart attack or calcification risk. If you are personally concerned about this topic, I recommend listening to Dave Feldman and even using his cholesterol calculator. It can usually be found on cholesterolcode.com; however, you can always access the direct link through our resources page at ReversingPKD.com/resources This will give you a far better insight into your actual disease risk. Some simple insights can be gained from your:

- HDL: (high is good; 50-80 is usually a good place for keto dieters)
- HDL/triglyceride ratio: (you want your HDL to be higher than your triglycerides)
- Remnant cholesterol: (total cholesterol minus HDL minus LDL, at most should be 15; mine is zero).

So why are our reference ranges for cholesterol so low and how can it be okay to be over the range for some of these values? The answer is that these reference ranges have been conceived by averaging out cholesterol levels over the (averagely sick) population. Now, the population has been told to eat a low-fat diet and focus mostly on unsaturated fats. This way of eating naturally lowers cholesterol levels, which is not a good thing. You can think of cholesterol as a team of firefighters. If you were an alien coming to earth for the first time and you saw a bunch of burning buildings, and every time there was a burning building you saw firefighters at the scene, you might start thinking to yourself that these firefighters might be responsible for the fire. Nothing could be further from the truth, however.

Whenever there's inflammation in your body, which corresponds to the fire in our example, your body sends cholesterol to repair the inflamed area, such as in your arteries.

Now usually the inflammation would slowly subside, the body would rebuild the damaged tissues and no further cholesterol would appear at the site. Nowadays, however, most people keep constantly triggering inflammation, mostly by eating processed junk and inflammatory oxidized omega-6 seed oils, so cholesterol keeps piling up at the site. Only after a ridiculously long amount of time does this start to become an issue. So it's not about the cholesterol; it's about the inflammation that we need to quench. Anybody adhering to the PKDproof program will not be having this issue any longer.

You can even monitor and measure your progress by getting regular CAC (coronary artery calcium) scans and noting the progress in your calcium score. Please do not be fooled by the clean results on your coronary ultrasound. This does not show actual plaque build-up; it only shows the empty space in between artery walls. If there's plaque inside your artery walls, which is very common, it will not be visible.

When we take a closer look at elevated triglyceride levels, it makes sense to take into account animal protein intake. Elevated levels of triglycerides, especially on a low-animal-protein diet, have been linked to creatine deficiency. Creatine is a conditionally essential nutrient, which means we can't produce enough of it inside the body. It is made up of amino acids and plays a crucial part in cell energy metabolism. Supplementing with creatine, or even better, getting it from animal foods like beef or clean fish, has been shown to reduce triglyceride levels substantially.[3]

Phosphate and potassium

Track your levels of phosphate and potassium as these electrolytes can get elevated in later stages of PKD in some people. Adjustments can be made to lower your levels – see Chapter 6: Adjustments for low kidney function on page 73.

Hemoglobin

Some PKD patients can see their iron and hemoglobin levels decrease with disease progression, and severe cases of anemia are actually treated with EPO (erythropoetin) injections. This is definitely something to look into when your levels are low; however, please do the basics first and make sure that you are eating ample amounts of red meat because it contains the most bioavailable form of iron, called heme-iron, which in and of itself can be enough to alleviate some cases of anemia. Absorption is paramount.

Iron deficiency can also be a symptom of copper deficiency. More info on this can also be found in Chapter 6: Adjustments for low kidney function.

Fasting insulin

Getting a fasting insulin test done every now and then is also a good idea. Just like fasting blood sugar, fasting insulin can be elevated even when you're on a ketogenic diet. This is an even more sensitive marker for insulin resistance and possibly beta-cell dysfunction. In some cases, even when fasting blood sugar is normal, fasting insulin can be high (above 4 uUL/ml). If you discover this, consider adding more carb days, or more carbs to your carb days if you were still holding back a bit.

If that's still not enough, take a look at your hip to waist ratio. If that is not optimal, just continue on the program until you see an improvement there. If that's not it, just as with fasting blood sugar, take a look at your stress levels using a morning cortisol or DUTCH test with a qualified practitioner.

Ferritin

As we already discussed earlier (page 84), ferritin, measured in serum is actually not something that should be present in the amounts we usually see today. Ferritin belongs inside the cell and any ferritin outside the cell is a sign of a certain degree of cell damage or inflammation. Contrary to popular belief, a level of ferritin below 40 is a good sign in healthy people. Of course there are more complex considerations as it can also be low because of an actual iron deficiency, so this is an important distinction to understand.

When ferritin levels are high and you don't have any issue with anemia, regular blood donations are a good strategy to lower the iron burden on your body. Men actually have no way to get rid of excess iron, contrary to women who lose some every month until menopause. After that they can also benefit from regular blood donations. This is an essential anti-aging strategy.

To learn more about why ferritin and other common markers for iron status, such as TIBC and transferrin saturation, are much more complex and highly influenced by bioavailable copper status, I recommend reading the fascinating *Root Cause Protocol* blog by Morley Robbins.[4]

That said, if your iron status as a whole is low, blood donations are not for you.

Thyroid hormones

Nowadays we have an epidemic of thyroid dysfunction, and most of it is actually Hashimoto's thyroiditis, which means an autoimmune attack on the thyroid gland, resulting in low levels of thyroid hormone and elevated levels of TSH (thyroid stimulating hormone). In many cases, antibody levels are also elevated, but this isn't always measurable. The thyroid can be thought of as being like your body's master thermostat, and when that is turned down, nothing really works as it should. This can be a major impediment to healing, so it should not be overlooked.

A basic 'thyroid panel' (suite of tests) should include at the very least TSH, FT3 (free triiodothyronine) and FT4 (free thyroxine). The TSH result will tell you the level of thyroid stimulating hormone, which is produced by the pituitary gland. This is the hormone your body uses to tell your thyroid that it needs to make more hormone. If FT3 or FT4 levels are low, TSH levels go up. It is helpful to know your TSH level from early on, so you have something to compare your current levels with when you suspect dysfunction. Everybody's different, so reference ranges have to be taken with a pinch of salt. That said, any TSH above 2 mU/l should give you pause and might indicate that your FT3 or FT4 thyroid hormones might be lower than they should be.

FT3 and FT4 levels need to be analyzed in conjunction. FT4 is the actual hormone that your thyroid makes out of iodine, while FT3 is the hormone that is converted throughout your body from FT4. The ratio of these two hormones can therefore tell us a lot about production and conversion and can give us a hint about where an issue might lie. Pay attention to the units that your lab measures them in and convert them if necessary. The functional reference ranges, meaning the reference ranges for optimal health, vary slightly between practitioners but one example is the functional range by Dr Bruce Rind, MD:[5]

- FT3: 2.3–4.2 pg/ml
- FT4: 0.8–1.8 ng/dl

You want both of your results to lie somewhere in that range, preferably around the middle; however, the most important thing to pay attention to is how far into the range each of your results is. You want both to be no more than 5% different from each other. So for example, if your FT4 was at a level of 1.2 ng/dl, that's 33% of the range, so you'd expect your FT3 to be somewhere between 28-38% into the range, so between 3.42 pg/ml and 3.57 pg/ml. Anything below that shows a conversion issue, while everything higher than that shows a production issue.

The easiest way to remedy many cases of conversion trouble is by supplementing with 200 grams of sodium selenite per day, and the easiest way to remedy many cases of production trouble is by supplementing with up to 3000 mg clean kelp powder or even a couple of drops of Lugol's iodine per day. Your need and tolerance for iodine are very individual, so try to see how you feel on it and intermittently try the iodine patch test; this entails using Lugol's to paint a 3 x 3 inch (7.5 x 7.5 cm) square on your abdomen, inner thigh or inner forearm and then seeing how long the yellow staining takes to disappear. This shows if you are still deficient – if it's still there after 24 hours, you are probably not iodine deficient; if it disappears more quickly than that, iodine supplementation is probably for you.

Stool testing

If we want to address endotoxin (see page 30), as a first step it is probably a good idea to get checked for any kind of gut dysbiosis as it is the gut bacteria manufacturing most of our endotoxin burden.

One option would be to use a VIOME stool test, which you can easily order online. This test can help to improve the makeup of your gut flora and even reduce the number of endotoxin-producing gram-negative bacteria that are present. They list endotoxin-producing bacteria on the results page and give actionable insights into which foods to limit and which ones to boost to lower your level of some of these unwanted gut inhabitants.

Imaging (MRI, CT, ultrasound)

The most accurate way to predict PKD progression is to track kidney volume over time. While there are several options for doing this, MRI is the gold standard. Ultrasound can be very unreliable regarding accurate tracking of cyst size or kidney length, much less kidney volume. However, even MRI is usually not used to make super-accurate calculations since nobody is really taking the time to calculate the kidney volume accurately. Instead, they use an ellipsoid calculation which is basically just taking some crude measurements of kidney length and diameter and then applying those to an ellipsoid shape, which is then used to estimate kidney volume.

You could pay someone to make a much more accurate calculation from the MRI images, but this is usually not done by doctors or MRI technicians. Actually looking at the images side-by-side, in addition to whatever volume was calculated, may give you a more complete understanding of your progression.

When trying to measure exact changes in PKD kidneys following an extreme regimen, a PET-CT scan can also be of value, as it can show fermentation activity directly, like lights on a Christmas tree. This way you can even distinguish between living and dead tissue. However, this will cause additional radiation exposure from either the injected liquid, the scan itself or both, which can lead to injury, so use with caution.

Chapter 11

What to do regularly

So, as we are trying to do what was previously thought impossible here, let's quickly take a look at all the methods we have to do the following:

- Maximize autophagy (damaged cell clean up) during fasting
- Minimize and target growth to occur in the right tissues during feeding.

Maximizing autophagy

Intermittent fasting

Intermittent fasting (IF), also sometimes, and more accurately, called 'time-restricted eating' or TRE, is one of the ways we can turbo-charge ketone production as well as autophagy. It will also go a long way to inhibiting mTOR at night and is the basis for our strategy. While exact numbers on fasting durations are hard to come by, researchers are pretty sure that autophagy genes begin to get upregulated somewhere between the 15- and 18-hour fasting marks. Individual fitness level measured by VO_2 max is a large influence on this too, as we discussed earlier (page 20). Anything over 18 hours of fasting will likely interfere with proper nutrient absorption, and while some people swear by the 'one meal a day' (OMAD) regimen, I believe this makes it far too difficult to absorb as many nutrients as we need, especially considering the state of our food supply these days. Our food is not nearly as nutrient-dense as it used to be only a couple of decades ago, so quantity matters even if you're getting very high-quality vegetables and animal products.

Also, especially in the later stages of PKD, we need to make sure that every gram of protein is absorbed optimally since we are going to filter its nitrogen components regardless. Consequently, it makes sense to space out meals as widely as possible within the eating window, which would at the minimum be six hours long. It makes sense to move this window to an earlier spot in the day so that you can get two to four hours fasting in before you go to bed to give your body and brain a chance to focus on cleaning and repair during the night rather than digesting food.

This is more important than many people realize. A couple of years ago scientists discovered a mechanism by which our bodies clean up proteins and debris from our brains during sleep; it's called the 'glymphatic system'. It sounds very similar to the 'lymphatic system', and that's because it is. It's simply the lymphatic system in the brain rather than in the rest of the body, but its purpose is the same. That is, to get rid of waste, by pumping cerebrospinal fluid through the brain tissues, and to keep our brains young and healthy in the process. This system mainly works in deep sleep and requires a lot of blood flow, which is disturbed by late-night meals sucking all the blood away to your stomach for digestion. So, keep your eating window at least two, optimally four, hours away from bedtime if you can. This way you will be optimizing recovery in all areas of your body, which is exactly what the doctor ordered. Or at least what you want.

Intermittent fasting in this way will also give your body an even better chance at producing its own ketones, as this is evolutionarily how we kept going when there was no food around. In addition, the body will also start looking for damaged proteins anywhere it can to make up for the lack of protein intake in the fasting period. This is great news because cells expressing the PKD mutation are more likely to be damaged and so they have a greater likelihood of getting recycled into their raw materials and finally made into new, healthy cells.

Water fasting

While water fasting is a popular strategy that is touted by many health advocates, full-on water fasting does have severe downsides, especially for people with detox impairments such as PKD patients.

Whenever you fast, your body begins the process of lipolysis, meaning the breakdown of fat cells, which then release stored energy in the form of fatty acids. Now, since our bodies also store toxins inside fat cells to protect us from anything our bodies can't readily excrete, these toxins are released as well. Usually most toxins get excreted into the gut and they slowly move out. In water fasting, there just is not enough movement in the gut to get rid of these toxins, so the body reabsorbs, and redistributes, them, leading to possible toxin redistribution issues.

In short, water fasting used to be a great strategy when the Earth was a less toxic place, but nowadays toxins are so ubiquitous we need to adjust this strategy to do less harm than good. It's a much better idea to do protein fasting as described next.

Protein fasting

Protein fasting is a great addition to an intermittent fasting regime for anyone who has PKD to do about once a week; for the less physically fit it is paramount to do it for three to four consecutive days per month since they need much longer fasting periods to tap into mTOR inhibition and autophagy. Protein fasting this way enables us to excrete toxins while keeping mTOR activation to a minimum. Slowly work up to the multiple-day protocol if you need to.

This protein fast is a simplified version of Dr Mercola's *Ketofast*, which is a great book that goes into much more detail on the benefits of a modified fast like this.[2] A proper protein fast means you are not consuming more than 15 grams of protein or carbs on any given day and calculate the calories needed to optimally process toxins in this extreme detox period.

A small number of calories is essential even in a modified fast as they provide the energy required for the body to function optimally and to process toxins effectively during this extreme detox period. A calculated caloric intake ensures that the body has enough energy to support the detoxification processes without overwhelming the system, allowing for a smoother and more manageable fasting experience.

Fats play a pivotal role in this modified fast. They become the primary source of energy as the body transitions from burning glucose to burning fats. High-quality fats are crucial as they not only provide sustained energy but also aid the absorption of fat-soluble vitamins, which are vital for overall health and wellbeing during the fasting period.

Bone broth also plays an important role in maintaining your tissues during a fast, but it does not activate mTOR and therefore keeps autophagy going. During a protein fast, especially one that spans multiple days, it's essential to monitor weight loss closely. If you lose excessive weight (more than 3-4 pounds – that's 1.36-1.8 kg), it's sensible to increase the intake of collagen from sources like bone broth to more than the initial 15 grams, potentially doubling or even tripling it if necessary. This adjustment is particularly crucial during multiple-day protein fasts.

Now for the calculations; we will look at how to find out your body fat percentage, so you can calculate your lean body mass next.

Protein fasting calculations

To calculate your calorie needs on protein fasting days, we first need to estimate your body fat percentage (BFP). If you want to do these calculations for yourself, and enjoy the math, I've included what is known as the 'Relative Fat Mass formula' below. Most readers will probably want to use the online calculator at www.ReversingPKD.com/report. You can also use a body fat scale for a rough estimate; however, this will be less accurate.

We can estimate our body fat percentage from measuring our waist circumference. For this, use a flexible measuring tape to measure around your body at the level of the top of the left and right ilium on the hip (the largest and highest bone in the hip). Take the measurement at the peak of an exhale, which will be the smallest measurement.

Estimate body fat percentage (BFP):
For men: BFP = 64 - (20 x [height/waist circumference])
For women: BFP = 76 - (20 x [height/waist circumference])

Once you know your body fat percentage, you also know your lean mass, which is the remainder. So, for example, for a 150-pound (68 kg) human with 15% body fat, lean body mass would be 85%, so:

0.85 x 150 lb = 127.5 lb

Then you can calculate your calorie needs for protein fasting days like this:

3.5 x (your lean body weight in pounds)

So calorie needs for protein fasting in our 150-pound example would be:

3.5 x 127.5 = 446.25 kcal.

Practically speaking, since you will begin the day with a bulletproof coffee, you can subtract its calories from the total calories that remain for lunch. Every gram of fat represents 9 kcal.

With 15 g MCT oil and 15 g butter, that gives us a total of 270 kcal in one cup of bulletproof coffee.

So for lunch in our example there would be 176 kcal left to budget.

To make it really easy then, you can just choose a non-starchy vegetable, see how much of it you can fit into the carbohydrate and calorie budget, and fill the rest with bone broth until you hit your protein target. Of course you can make other recipes as well, there's even Dr. Mercola's cookbook just for these protein-fasting days – *The Ketofast Cookbook* – if you need more ideas.[2] But, for this example, roughly 150 g Brussels sprouts and 150 ml bone broth would hit the target almost exactly. Your mileage may vary.

I recommend using the free app 'Cronometer' to track your food intake in the first couple of weeks anyway, so this is a great opportunity to put in the protein fasting day foods in advance. This way you can be sure that your macronutrients check out. You can find a couple more meal suggestions later in this book (page 227).

You can use your protein fast to incorporate some glutamine-inhibiting strategies like the supplements or medications discussed earlier. It is in the protein fast that your ketones will be at their highest, glucose will be at its lowest and the body will be scouring for extra protein. If you give the PKD cells the extra 'pulse' of restricting their glutamine emergency fuel (see page 16), you will make it much more likely for these cells to be dissolved and used as a source of building blocks for the rest of the body ('autolytic cannibalism').

Coffee

Contrary to popular belief, coffee is not contraindicated in PKD. As we mentioned before (page 102), this common misconception has been disproven by several studies.[3] In short, it makes sense to measure your blood pressure before and after consuming some caffeinated coffee and see if there is a significant difference. If there is not, you can drink coffee. If there is a significant jump, try decaf.

However, as I have emphasized before, you will want to make sure that your coffee is tested for mold toxins, which is one of the most pervasive issues in coffee production worldwide. There are a couple of brands that advertise lab-tested coffee beans; the most extensive testing seems to be done by the 'Bulletproof' brand.

Some key points to remember are: there are two active methylxanthines in coffee, caffeine and theophylline, which are highly effective mTOR inhibitors. In addition, coffee is also effective in stimulating the limited flow of Ca^{2+}, which is an issue in PKD. Add to this all the extra benefits of putting butter and MCT oil in your coffee and that's a powerful combination.

High-intensity repeat training (HIRT)

You may already have heard about high-intensity interval training, or HIIT. While this is a very popular and effective way to train, for individuals with health challenges like diabetes, or heart disease, it may not be the most suitable form of exercise.

Specifically, research has indicated that HIIT can pose elevated risks for individuals with underlying health conditions such as diabetes and heart disease. A study published in the *World Journal of Cardiology* found that engaging in HIIT might increase the likelihood of cardiac events in people with pre-existing heart conditions.[4] It might also not be suited to diabetics, increasing cardiac risks.[5] If you are type 2 diabetic, a couple of months on the Bulletproof Diet might solve that issue for you (though even type-1s can greatly reduce their insulin usage on this diet).

HIRT (high-intensity *repeat* training) improves on HIIT by allowing for longer rest periods between high-intensity repeats, reducing overall fatigue and requiring less recovery time after the session. This approach ensures that people do not overexert themselves, avoiding excessive energy depletion that can aggravate health conditions like diabetes, or heart disease.

HIRT provides a superior and sustainable way to engage in high-intensity workouts safely, while being even more effective.[6] That said, if you are pressed for time in your lunch break and you are not diabetic and have no pre-existing heart disease, it can make sense to reduce the recovery times to a traditional HIIT session in your individual case. In that case, probably it's better to do HIIT if there is not enough time to do HIRT.

Heavy weights

I recommend doing a HIRT weight-training session in a fasted state once per week, which means you are going to be lifting heavy things, meaning about 80% of the maximum weight you could lift. If you feel energetic in the mornings even without bulletproof coffee, you can go ahead and do a completely fasted workout, but if you feel in your workout you are missing energy, then go ahead and drink a cup of bulletproof coffee beforehand so you have a ketone boost for your workout.

With all exercise, you have to keep in mind that once energy demands are high enough, your body will begin producing glucose from your muscles. This process is called gluconeo-genesis. So this means when you overexert yourself for an extended period of time, this can actually raise your blood glucose level, which gives PKD cells more raw materials to accelerate their growth, similar to a carb day. Luckily you will be in a fasted state and therefore mTOR will be low, but it's a much better idea to control your exercise in a way that will not cross this threshold whenever you want to maximize the mTOR-inhibiting effects of your fast. Enter **MAF heart-rate training**.

This is a pretty simple concept: you calculate your maximum heart rate by subtracting your age from 180. So, if you are 50 years old, your MAF heart rate will be 130. If in your training routine you exceed your MAF heart rate, your body will begin producing glucose from your muscles to keep up with energy demands. As long as you stay below this threshold, your body will be able to meet energy demands by metabolizing ketones. Training below MAF heart rate for an extended period of time will train your body to be more efficient with its ketone use. This will enable you to go for much longer without eating since you can metabolize the enormous amount of energy from fat that is stored on your body, instead of the measly 2000 calories or less that are in your glycogen stores. If you are a runner, it will also enable you to run faster and faster with time without breaching your threshold, since this way you will actually be training the aerobic part of your mitochondrial metabolism.

Now the simple form of HIRT using machines in the gym will likely not make you exceed your MAF heart rate, since it is taking place in very short bursts with large rest periods in between that allow you to recover completely. You can find a video of the recommended training method on my YouTube channel and website www.ReversingPKD.org, but we will look at a basic regimen next. In the unlikely event that your heart rate does increase enough to be above MAF heart rate, adjust timing, duration or intensity accordingly. If this doesn't work, or you want to do high heart rate exercise, it can make sense to move your exercise regimen to your eating window, optimally on carb refeed days.

Sample workout

So, keeping with the considerations we talked about earlier, here's one example of a workout that is optimized for building muscle, recycling damaged cells and keeping glucose production to a minimum for PKD benefits. The following machines are the 'big five', as coined by Dr Doug McGuff. All of these are so-called 'compound movements', meaning they don't isolate any single muscle group and instead require multiple muscle groups at the same time to perform the movement.

- Seated row
- Chest press
- Pulldown
- Overhead press
- Leg press.

On each of these machines, you would first find the weight that you can slowly move up and down again once within 10 to 15 seconds. It is important these movements be very slow so we give the body a chance to run on the more efficient, but slower ketone metabolism – that is, 5 seconds up, 5 seconds down… or longer. You should be able to do this six to eight times in a row with 1 minute of complete rest in between. However, the movement must be smooth. If it becomes jerky, you need to increase the speed until it gets smooth again and do more movements in your time interval. It might take you one or two training days to figure out which is your optimal weight so you can actually complete the movement enough times, but not more. Please make sure to keep your head straight at all times and, if you cannot move the weight as much as you would like, hold it instead of shifting around to try to get it to move a little more. Form is important.

Immediately after your exercise is when you break your fast. Optimally you would have a protein-rich lunch up to an hour after finishing your training. You can also have a grass-fed whey protein shake to increase your protein intake after your workout.

Studies have shown that an intense training session like this will target mTOR activation towards the muscle[7] and therefore give you less of a growth response in glycolytic tissues like tumors and, by extension, cysts than you would expect on a day without exercise.

Cardio

For all the runners out there, it can require some adaptation to adjust your regimen to be optimal for reversing PKD. Most runners train close to their maximum heart rate, which, as we discussed, pushes the body into anaerobic metabolism. This increases blood glucose as the body rapidly ramps up glycolysis, which of course is not what we want in PKD. Therefore, for anyone who's not going to give up their maximum heart rate training regimen, it would be best to do it on carb days and definitely in the eating window.

If you're not a runner yet, or you are interested in designing a running routine that actually increases mitochondrial function and therefore the body's capability to use oxygen (which might even benefit PKD), this is the ticket. Just as in strength training, MAF heart rate (180 minus your age) can also be used for running, building up VO_2 max through purely aerobic exercise. This type of running can usually be done in ketosis and even in the fasting window if desired.

When you do this regularly, your mitochondria's capability to use oxygen for energy will steadily increase, mirrored by faster times for the same distance at your MAF heart rate. In the beginning this can be a very slow pace as your mitochondria start to get used to working at their maximum and build up higher capacity.

The exercise period can be increased according to your personal progress, but it is fine to start with just five minutes for beginners, in addition to the warm-up and cool-down periods, which should be about one-third as long as your workout period respectively. A basic exercise outline might look like this:

- 12 minutes warm-up: gradually increase your heart rate from resting to just below your MAF heart rate, giving you a bit of a buffer.
- up to 45 minutes exercise at or slightly below your MAF heart rate, increasing duration according to your progress.
- 12 minutes cool-down: gradually decrease your heart rate from MAF to resting by slowing your pace.

A shorter routine could be 2 minutes warm-up, 5 minutes at MAF heart rate, 2 minutes cool-down and so on.

Medical doctor and running enthusiast Peter Attia suggests a total of 2-3 hours' running per week as the minimum effective dose for increasing performance in actual runners.[8] So, you could do a running workout like this two or three times a week to go all-out, or you could do whatever short routine fits your schedule. This is very individual. As long as your time per mile keeps decreasing, you are making progress towards a higher VO_2 max and better health.

Another option would be a HIRT sprint workout that keeps sprinting intervals around 10 seconds, which is about the time your body needs to deplete energy reserves stored as ATP. This is called the 'alactic system' as no lactate is produced in the process. With generous recovery times of 1-5 minutes in between, depending on your state of fitness, you will train your cardiovascular system without the need for switching energy metabolism to glycolysis. This can be a quicker form of exercise, but you will miss out on the benefits of training more efficient mitochondria, which, as we have discussed earlier, are a main area of focus in PKD.

Minimizing growth

Supplements for minimizing growth

Multi-talents

Exogenous ketones

Higher blood levels of ketones have been shown to upregulate our ability to detox endotoxin (see page 30), so in addition to nutritional ketosis, supplementation with MCT oil, or possibly even exogenous ketones like BHB salts, or optimally ketone esters, is a good idea. However, the content of racemic, meaning 'not biologically identical ketones', in most ketone salts makes them a suspect supplement. There have been researchers concerned with their potential as a mitochondrial toxin. A safer option might be so-called D-BHB, which only contains the bioidentical form of the ketone BHB. However, even those need to be considered with caution, as you will be taking in lots of minerals in the process, so find out what your levels are and possibly talk to your doctor about it.

The safest, most effective and most expensive option would be exogenous ketone esters, which don't contain any minerals and can get your ketone levels far higher than any other supplement. They're a very interesting option for sure and you don't need much of them. The most popular brand is called KetoneAid and is available online.

Polyphenols

Polyphenols are Mother Nature's autophagy enhancers. When you take them in your fasting window, mTOR inhibition goes even higher and they do seem to potentiate each other's effects. You can choose to take a couple of capsules, which is convenient, or you can decide to go the Autophagy tea route (page 234), which is more affordable and comprehensive.

One of the most well-known and effective polyphenols on the

market today is quercetin. It is a yellow-colored plant flavonol that can be extracted from Japanese knotweed rhizomes; however, is it also found in common foods like onions, apples, blueberries and broccoli, as well as honey. Quercetin, like many of the polyphenol family, is a potent mTOR inhibitor and therefore improves the effects of fasting. In a 2017 study on a PKD mouse model, researchers injected the mice with quercetin and saw a roughly 30% reduction in cyst growth rate.[9] The human equivalent dose for this study would probably be around 5 grams of quercetin per day, but there aren't conclusive safety studies on dosages as high as this. Limited evidence from animal studies suggests that existing kidney damage and estrogen-dependent cancers could be risk factors, but in humans quercetin has actually been shown to be kidney protective and cancer protective.[10]

Safety studies testing up to 5 grams in humans per day haven't shown any toxicity, a standard dose being between 1 and 2 grams per day. So somewhere between 1 and 5 grams per day[11, 12] might be the sweet spot for now.

Quercetin and fisetin have also both been shown to be quite potent at upregulating an enzyme called argininosuccinate synthase, which is giving us more protection from endotoxin and inhibiting glycolysis, but they are even stronger when we combine them with arginine's precursor citrulline, which I'll address in the next section on endotoxin mitigators.

Milk thistle

Milk thistle is a very popular supplement in the anti-aging space, as it upregulates liver detox enzymes and thereby increases resistance to endotoxin. However, it should be noted that milk thistle should only be taken intermittently, so one month on, one month off would be a good starting point, to prevent any kind of tolerance effect.

You can either take it with food to help your liver with digestion or you can take it at night as an extra mTOR inhibitor.

Endotoxin mitigators

Citrulline

So we talked about the fact that – genetically – PKD patients have low levels of argininosuccinate synthase (AS), the enzyme needed to make argininosuccinate. So you might now assume that supplementing extra argininosuccinate could have a benefit, right? If we can't make enough, let's put more into the system? Well, not so fast. It's not the argininosuccinate itself we are interested in; it is the enzyme that makes it.

Interestingly, studies have shown that, the more argininosuccinate is removed, the more AS is upregulated. When we think about this, it does make sense. When we have less of something, the body will probably try to upregulate the process that produces more of it. More AS means more protection from endotoxin. More AS also means more inhibition of glycolysis, which means less cyst growth.

However, removing argininosuccinate from the kidney is not something that can be easily achieved without pharmaceuticals, so we should probably look at other ways to change this balance.

If one scenario where AS gets upregulated is when it senses low argininosuccinate, another scenario might be when it senses that there is too much citrulline – the amino acid that AS converts to argininosuccinate – as it's all about the ratio between the two. This gives our body the signal that there is too much citrulline to be metabolized by current levels of AS, which can be done synergistically with quercetin and fisetin, as they upregulate the correlating gene expression in kidney cells to make more AS effectively.

The combination of fisetin and citrulline in one study[13] was stronger than each of them separately, suggesting a synergistic effect. Adding some more quercetin to this is probably a good idea, since it has a similar mechanism to fisetin, albeit a bit less strong. Think of it as the budget version.

Even citrulline alone in one study on a mouse model of sepsis (lots of endotoxin in the blood) increased arginine and restored T-cell mitochondrial function while reducing the effects of endotoxin.[14]

As two additional benefits, citrulline supplementation has been shown to lower blood pressure and upregulate AS and it also seems to improve the preservation of the inner layer of the colon, contributing to keeping the bad guys out of our bloodstream.

While dosing considerations are theoretical at this point, one study on cyclists' performance enhancement used a 2.4-gram dose per day.[15] Citrulline can lower blood pressure as well, so start low and slow. A 2017 study assessing the safety of citrulline concluded it was safe even for critically ill patients.[16] One trial actually showed it as being kidney protective for diabetic mice.[17]

If you are limiting protein, keep in mind that supplementing citrulline counts towards your protein intake, or rather your nitrogen budget since it is an amino acid. Citrulline is an mTOR activator, so it should be taken in the eating window.

Probiotics

An interesting way to decrease the production of endotoxin straight out of the gate would be to take a probiotic called Megasporebiotic. One study in people with high blood endotoxin levels after a meal showed that Megaspore could reduce it by 42%.[18] While this one usually needs to be ordered through a practitioner, some websites still offer it for sale online. I also order it for my clients; you can visit www.ReversingPKD.com if you are interested in working with me directly. A good starting dosage is two capsules with a meal, just as stated on the package.

Many other probiotics can be used to reduce endotoxin levels, and while details go beyond the scope of this book, they include:

- *Lactobacillus casei*

- *Lactobacillus subtilis*
- *Lactobacillus acidophilus*
- *Lactobacillus lactis*
- *Bifidobacterium animalis*
- Spore-based probiotics
- VSL#3

Getting a VIOME stool test can give you a good idea of which strains would most benefit your individual gut makeup and reduce your endotoxin producers.

Charcoal and chitosan

Activated charcoal and chitosan are potent adsorbents for different toxins, including endotoxin, and can be a great choice for a nighttime supplement. Since food has already been digested then, as long as there are no medications that have to be taken at this time, they are free to bind toxins in the body, including endotoxin in the gut as well as in the bloodstream.

Taking these won't actually increase autophagy by itself, but it is an important alternative approach to the nighttime supplement that we can take. Many of the initial injuries that are suspected to first trigger cyst growth might be attributable to toxins, so it only makes sense to consider mopping up some of the toxins in our bodies before they even reach the kidneys, or liver for that matter. As charcoal is a very potent adsorbent, it should only be taken two hours away from all food and supplements since it will inhibit the absorption of those too.

Chitosan is made from the shells of certain insects and preferentially binds lipids, meaning fats, but it also binds endotoxin. Some research suggests it's also possible to reduce blood urea nitrogen (BUN) levels, as well as increase glomerular filtration rates (GFR), by binding up toxins with chitosan, and most likely charcoal as well. One study in patients with chronic renal failure showed significant reductions in serum urea and creatinine levels after chitosan supplementation.[19] (See also page 79.) The average BUN dropped by 40% and creatinine dropped by 13% after 12 weeks of supplementing with 1.3 grams of chitosan three times per day.

The mechanism behind this was not clear to the researchers, though. Might there be an endotoxin connection behind this effect?

Other options with good efficacy include modified citrus pectin (MCP) and even cholestyramine, which is prescription-only and binds toxins in bile. Bile is otherwise a dead end for persisting toxins as it gets recycled indefinitely by the body. Most cholestyramine products on the market include unwanted additives, so getting a prescription for the pure powder and making your own capsules with a cheap capsule maker is by far the best option.

Prebiotics

Improving your gut flora with prebiotics has been shown to reduce the levels of endotoxin in several studies. Prebiotics that have shown good effectiveness include inulin, oligofructose, Sunfiber[20] and arabinogalactans,[21] which I talk about in detail a bit later, on page 157.

L-Glutamine

As you have surely gleaned from our discussion before, glutamine is a double-edged sword. It's the emergency fuel for PKD cells, fueling their growth even when glucose is low. On the other hand, it's a vital component of a healthy immune system, for muscle growth, the integrity of the gut lining and so much more. While it is not known to what degree the tight junctions lining the gut of PKD patients are compromised and how much of that is part of the disease progression and injury and how much is existing from birth, it is certainly a good idea to minimize the permeability of one's gut lining with some basic strategies. Before we consider any kind of supplementation to enhance the strength of our tight junctions, we have to make sure we are not doing anything to increase permeability, so therefore it is very important we limit our intake of lectins (page 43) from food.

Getting the VIOME stool test mentioned before (page 126) and adhering to the personalized food recommendations will also go a long way to ensuring the health of your intestinal lining. I would recommend you skip any foods from the bad zone of the Bulletproof Diet food list, even if they are recommended on your VIOME test results.

Once you have made sure that you are not jeopardizing the tightness of your tight junctions more than necessary, you can proceed to a protocol for repair. This probably will not repair any genetic leaky gut stemming from the PKD mutation, but it would at least get you back to your personal baseline, and that is probably more than can be said for most of the population.

A protocol like this might also increase blood glutamine levels temporarily and slightly, which could give some extra fuel to PKD cells for a short period of time, similar to a carbohydrate binge. However, it has the potential to heal your gut lining and therefore prevent further injury of the kidneys, so it's likely to be worth it.

L-Glutamine is one of the 20 amino acids that our body can use and in this context you can think of it as sort of the basic nutrition for the cells in your gut lining. When these cells get an adequate supply, they rapidly repair and regrow themselves. One protocol for this was developed by a world-class athletic trainer called Poliquin. His goal with this protocol was to ensure that athletes would be able to absorb as much of their nutrient intake as possible. His protocol can be regarded as a little bit heavy-handed, and he did have different goals than we do, so here's a modified, lighter version of it:

Over three days, work up to a dose of 30 grams of pure L-glutamine powder per day, divided evenly over all the meals in your eating window.

Stay at 30 grams per day for five days, then gradually taper off to 5 grams per day over the course of 10 days.

You might choose to stay at 5 grams per day for an extended period, or you might choose to stop the protocol; this entirely depends on your personal experience. Take note of any changes in your digestion, feeling of fullness, nausea, etc.

Remember, when you are on a protein-restricted diet, that glutamine is an amino acid and therefore counts towards your protein intake.

Collagen peptides

Collagen has been shown to improve the function of tight junctions by inhibiting the NFκB and ERK1/2 signaling pathways.[22] As a reminder, the tight junctions make up the continuous intercellular barrier among epithelial cells in the gut lining. These pathways are involved in the regulation of tight junction permeability and integrity, and interestingly they are also dysregulated in PKD.

In addition, collagen peptides were shown to prevent the breakdown of tight junction proteins and even reduce inflammation in the gut. They also contain many of the amino acids, such as glycine, needed in building tight junctions, so they might even aid their repair.[23]

mTOR inhibitors

Olive leaf extract

Some of the polyphenols found in olive oil can also be found in even higher concentrations in olive leaf and olive leaf extract, the most prevalent one being oleuropein.

Oleuropein has been shown to attenuate proliferation of cancer cells in numerous studies by activating AMPK and inhibiting mTOR. In a 2018 study it was also tested on PKD cell culture and indeed led to a reduction in cyst size.[24]

It is also a popular anti-aging supplement and easy to get in its powdered form; however, the much more bioavailable form is the liquid olive leaf extract in various formulations. Make sure to check for unwanted extra ingredients that might hide in the ingredients list when choosing a supplement brand. You can find brand recommendations on the resources page at ReversingPKD.com/resources.

Curcumin and ginkgo biloba

While curcumin (one of the main active substances in turmeric) and ginkgo biloba each on their own have potential to reduce cyst growth, when combined is when they really start to shine. In one study, the combination of both exhibited a greater effect on cyst growth than each of them separately so their effects are synergistic.[25] They hit a variety of different molecular pathways: upregulating intracellular calcium (Ca^{2+}), blocking MAPK, activating AMPK and inhibiting mTOR. You don't need to necessarily understand what all this means, just know it's probably a good idea to take the two supplements together.[26]

For ginkgo, you don't need any specific form, just one or two capsules of concentrated extract, 120 mg each, or some pure powdered extract will suffice.

Curcumin on the other hand needs to be in a specific form. I am advising against using powdered forms, especially the ones employing either piperine or black pepper as their absorption-enhancing additive. This includes capsules containing powder. You see, curcumin is not soluble in water and only ever so slightly in fat, so what manufacturers do is add something to increase the absorption into the bloodstream. When using black pepper or its extract, piperine, as well as some industrial absorption enhancers like polysorbate 80, this leads to the loosening of the tight junctions in our gut. This will increase the absorption of curcumin a little bit, but with it, everything else in the gut will be permeating into the bloodstream as well. This loosening, when present permanently, is also called 'leaky gut' and can give you a whole host of issues as we've seen, from all kinds of poisoning and infections through to triggering autoimmunity. So instead, I recommend finding a form of curcumin that uses other methods of increasing absorption, such as the 'black sludge' recipe later in this book (page 235). Commercially available forms that don't use black pepper or potentially toxic additives, at the time of going to press, are Theracurmin using nano-sized curcumin particles and Longvida using a lipid encapsulation. Longvida has better studies showing positive brain effects, while Theracurmin seems better suited for whole-body applications. You can find more brand recommendations on the book's resource page at ReversingPKD.com / resources.

Dosing can vary widely, but 300-600 mg daily from highly bioavailable sources is a good starting point.

Autophagy tea

Autophagy tea is a powerful combination of the well-established autophagy enhancers pau d' arco, garcinia, quercetin, glycine and chamomile. It's possibly the most effective and affordable way to trigger autophagy with supplement powders. Find the recipe on page 234.

Apple cider vinegar nighttime drink

Another simpler alternative to Autophagy tea is an apple cider vinegar-based nighttime drink, popularized by Thomas DeLauer. Simply take a cup of hot filtered water, add about 30 ml of apple cider vinegar, half a teaspoon of cinnamon, and liquid stevia to taste. This actually tastes pretty good and is a very warming and soothing drink to finish your evening. You can make it even more effective by swapping out the hot water with freshly brewed chamomile tea.

Apple cider vinegar boosts metabolic processes and speeds up the body's entry into autophagy. It lowers blood sugar levels and activates the AMPK pathway while inhibiting mTOR.

The addition of cinnamon is not just for flavor. It acts as an insulin imitator, stabilizing blood sugar levels further and avoiding disruptive spikes and crashes during the night. Furthermore, it activates the NRF2 pathway, promoting the creation of glutathione, which neutralizes free radicals, aids nighttime restoration and inhibits the mTOR pathway even more.

Liquid stevia sweetens the drink, offsetting the sour taste of the vinegar so we can avoid causing a spike in adrenaline levels, which is important for quick entry into ketosis. But not only that, steviol has actually been found to limit cyst growth in ADPKD via AMPK,[27] so it's a great addition to the drink by that fact alone.

Glycolysis blockers

Vitamin C

Vitamin C should be taken in the eating window (page 12) as it will break a fast. As discussed in Chapter 2, it can offset some glucose access for kidney cells and is good for general health and immunity. However, vitamin C's main component ascorbic acid has actually been vilified by some in the kidney health space out of a concern with potential kidney stone formation.

While high doses of synthetic ascorbic acid taken over a long period might be an issue, research on natural sources like rose hip extract indicates it can actually help prevent kidney stone formation. One study found that rose hip extract did not increase urine oxalate levels, which are the main concern of vitamin C critics; instead, it decreased kidney and urine calcium contents and even decreased the size and number of calcium oxalate stones in the kidneys. It also significantly increased the excretion of citrate, which is another important factor in preventing stone formation.[28] This suggests that whole-food sources of vitamin C, such as rose hips, may offer protective benefits against kidney stones, possibly due to the presence of co-factors that inhibit stone formation. Evidence shows 1000 mg (1 gram) of vitamin C from whole-food supplements like rose hips or acerola cherry is a good starting point.

Methylene blue

The chemical dye called methylene blue (MB) is one of the oldest organic dyes. In addition to its use as a blue coloring agent, it also has the unique property of being able to make cells in aerobic glycolysis revert back to their state of aerobic respiration by donating electrons to the electron transport chain. It has been shown that taking methylene blue for a longer period might be able to reverse tumor resistance to autophagy and get cells to revert to a healthy state of mitochondrial respiration.

Doses ranging from 0.5-4 mg/kg in humans have been shown to be safe and effective. Just make sure you don't stain your toilet bowl, as your pee will have a bluish green tint! One way to titrate your dosage optimally is to start low and then increase slowly over a couple of days until you first see urine discoloration. Then you step the dosage back to the previous day's level, which then will be your target amount.

Glutamine blockers

These strategies, contrary to the rest of this book, are not suited or intended to be used on an ongoing basis. Rather, they should at most be used intermittently if diet alone fails to produce tangible reductions in kidney volume. Mechanistically it is unclear whether these lead to an increase in kidney function or not, as the killing of cystic tissue itself would not necessarily improve the remaining nephrons' function. However, less cystic tissue also means less injury to – and structural blockage of – remaining functioning nephrons, making it a potential prevention and improvement strategy. These strategies are emerging in cancer management: four to six cycles of 21 days over a period of six months are common. Since PKD is a much slower progressing disease, these timings could potentially be a lot more relaxed, although this has to be assessed on an individual basis by following results via MRI, or even PET-CT scan, to make sure metabolically inactive ('dead') tissues can be detected after a cycle even if they still take up a similar amount of space.

Prescription drugs that lower glutamine levels include:
- DON (6-diazo-5-oxo-L-norleucine)
- Phenylbutyrate

Synergistic drugs include:
- Chloroquine
- Mebendazole and fenbendazole

Supplements that lower glutamine levels include:
- EGCG (epigallocatechin gallate, an extract from green tea)
- Curcumin
- Berberine.

Strenuous multi-hour anaerobic exercise and multiple-day fasting have also been found to decrease blood glutamine levels, as the body will convert part of it to glucose.[29] Creating higher glucose levels from glutamine may limit the efficacy of these methods, with fasting likely being the better choice as overall glucose will be lower on average in fasting compared to intense anaerobic exercise where glucose initially tends to increase.

The basic idea is to 'pulse' glutamine-inhibiting strategies during a period of particularly high ketosis, combined with oxidative therapy. For example, doing a session in a hyperbaric oxygen chamber (HBOT) during a single- or multiple-day protein fast, or a calorie-restricted diet with a high ratio of fat to protein-and-carbohydrate of about 2:1. The higher the ketones and the lower the glucose levels, the better.

The key factor to keep in mind is that, in cancer management, therapeutically low levels of glucose are in the 55-65 mg/dl range. These are paramount for glutamine-blocking strategies to have an effect. If glucose is higher, that is what cells with damaged mitochondria, as in cancer or PKD, will ferment to make energy using aerobic glycolysis. This has been repeatedly stated by Professor Thomas Seyfried in his research on metabolic therapies for cancer and very likely applies to PKD as well.

As glutamine cannot be inhibited much using diet, apart from extreme fasting, supplements and drugs become the only options to decrease blood levels of this vital amino acid to starve PKD cells just enough for them to die. All of these should be used in a 'pulse' strategy, giving the body time to recover in between. Note that the known effects of natural supplements on glutamine metabolism are still quite weak.

When cancer cells are experiencing the highest possible stress, being exposed to glucose and glutamine restriction simultaneously, in metabolic therapy for cancer usually a 90-minute session of HBOT inside a pressure chamber is administered. This exposes cells to high levels of reactive oxygen species, which then pushes them over the edge. It is very likely that this strategy works for PKD cells as well. Usually, a pressure of 2.75 atmospheres and 100% oxygen is used. Preliminary data in cancer suggests that 2 atmospheres of pressure might suffice, albeit requiring 50% more sessions for the same amount of reduction in tumor size.

DON (6-diazo-5-oxo-L-norleucine)

The glutamine analog DON (6-Diazo-5-oxo-L-norleucine), which was mentioned earlier, is the key pharmaceutical component of the metabolic cancer treatment protocols pioneered by Professor Thomas Seyfried. DON is structurally similar to glutamine, which allows it to interfere with the enzymes that normally use it. This is the strongest usable glutamine-inhibiting molecule known to date and it needs to be used very carefully, as side effects can be severe if administered or monitored incorrectly. The dosage regimen typically starts at 0.3 milligrams per kilogram of body weight and escalates up to 1.3 milligrams per kilogram over several months. It should be given with about 30 grams of fiber from finely ground psyllium husk to prevent severe gastrointestinal side effects. When administered correctly, in combination with having therapeutic levels of blood glucose, cancer cells are either killed or paralyzed, ready to be overloaded with oxygen during HBOT.

Sourcing and administration of DON can be a challenge and requires a detailed, meticulously timed strategy, as it requires rest days in between doses. **It should not be taken without medical supervision.**

Sodium phenylbutyrate

Sodium phenylbutyrate, after metabolism, binds glutamine in the blood. This complex is then excreted in urine, which reduces plasma glutamine levels. A study in humans showed that oral phenylbutyrate at a dosage of 0.36 g/kg/day led to a significant 26% decrease in plasma glutamine levels in healthy adults.[30] It is taken in tablet or powder form, with peak blood concentrations reached about one hour after ingestion, which is when any oxidative therapies like HBOT would be appropriate. The half-life is relatively short, so after approximately 45 minutes only half of the drug is left in the bloodstream. It's excreted through the kidneys, so if function is low, phenylbutyrate stays in the bloodstream for longer, meaning longer wait times between administrations would be appropriate.

Side effects, among others, can include gastrointestinal issues, electrolyte imbalance, headaches and fatigue.

Mebendazole and fenbendazole

While these are not directly blocking glutamine, mebendazole or fenbendazole usually are part of metabolic cancer treatment protocols because of their ability to inhibit glucose uptake and glycolytic enzymes. This creates a synergistic effect, as both glucose and glutamine pathways need to be blocked in cancer treatment. Mebendazole requires a prescription, while fenbendazole is available over-the-counter in some countries, albeit just offered for veterinary use.

Chloroquine

Chloroquine is often prescribed for prevention and treatment of malaria, but also used off-label for autoimmune issues. It enhances the efficacy of metabolic cancer treatment protocols by inhibiting lysosomal digestion, meaning it blocks the ability of the cell to ferment amino acids and carbohydrates gained from autophagy in the cells' immediate environment. Prescription is required.

EGCG

The natural green tea extract EGCG (epigallocatechin gallate), in addition to its capability to inhibit mTOR and activate autophagy, also has mild inhibitory effects on glutamine metabolism by lowering the activity of glutamate dehydrogenase 1 and 2. These are enzymes the body uses to make more glutamine from glutamate. A dosage regimen that has been used in cancer patients was 400 mg EGCG three times daily.[31] However, liver toxicity may become an issue at this point, so it is safer to keep it to around 400 mg/day, which in turn has been used in a cancer patient doing metabolic therapy.[32]

Curcumin

Curcumin has demonstrated potential in reducing glutamine availability through its ability to disrupt the transport of glutamine into cells, thus hindering their growth and survival. The mechanism likely involves the interaction of curcumin with cell membrane components or signaling pathways that regulate glutamine uptake. However, these effects are small and poorly documented. Therefore, adding standard doses to other glutamine-inhibiting strategies might be sensible.

Berberine

Berberine is an alkaloid found in several plants. It has been shown to inhibit the growth of liver cancer cells by suppressing glutamine uptake, as does curcumin. Consequently, it is very relevant in PKD. Berberine achieves this by down-regulating SLC1A5, a key transporter involved in cell glutamine uptake. By inhibiting SLC1A5, berberine reduces glutamine availability within the cancer cells, which is exactly what's needed in PKD. Berberine is used in mouse studies at dosages of around 5 mg/kg, which is quite low. Standard capsule sizes of 500 mg should therefore be a good starting point.[33] It also has slight beneficial effects on lowering blood glucose. Metabolic cancer therapies tend to use dosages of 1600-2000 mg per day.

Prebiotics

There is a human protein called galectin-3, a member of the lectin family. As we already discussed, lectins are bad news when it comes to health generally and also PKD specifically. Now for this particular lectin, there are some intriguing data that show higher levels are correlated with worse disease progression. This applies to general chronic kidney disease as well as PKD. One study in PKD patients showed there was a negative correlation between levels of serum galectin-3 and GFR levels, which are used to assess kidney function.[34] Luckily, there is a prebiotic that has been shown to bind to galectin-3.[35] It is a supplement called arabinogalactans, and you take a small scoop one to three times a day to maintain lower levels of galectin-3.

I also like to add some soluble SunFiber prebiotic (hydro-lyzed guar gum, see page 146) to sauces, meals or drinks as it is a tasteless water-soluble prebiotic that helps maintain a healthy gut flora.

Avoiding hidden sources of injury

We know that for most patients the PKD mutation is present in all kidney cells, but it only gets expressed whenever there is an additional injury to the cell that mutates the second copy of the gene, as was described at the start of the book (page 5). So, what constitutes an injury? Kidney cells can be injured by a variety of factors just like all cells in the body. It could be caused by stress, by an actual impact trauma like a car accident, by ionizing radiation from an international flight or by radioactive contrast enhancer for an MRI scan; even radiation from a regular CT (or CAT) scan could cause it. There is also the possibility of chemical injury – for example, from glyphosate or another pesticide/ herbicide. It could even be caused by additives and processed foods or toxic ingredients in beauty or personal care products like shampoos, shower gels, deodorants, lipsticks and so on. Even non-ionizing radiation from your phone or Wi-Fi could do it. So, it is paramount to limit your exposure to any of these sources of injury in all sensible ways that you can.

The Bulletproof Diet will take care of most of the foodborne toxins for you. By adhering to this way of eating, you will already have minimized your exposure to toxic pesticides, food additives, mold toxins and antinutrients. Now let's look at some other hidden sources of injury and what we can do about them.

Chemicals and everyday toxins

Toxic chemicals don't just come from food, so it is important for you to be mindful of your exposure to chemicals from all sources. These include, but are not limited to:

- Fragrances (think candles, detergents, perfumes, flavorings)
- Cleaning products (household cleaners, body hygiene products like shampoos, toothpaste and shower gels)
- Toxins in municipal water (chlorine, fluoride, traces of hormones and other medications)
- Medications.

For many of these you can find, or make, non-toxic alternatives:

- Shower gels and liquid hand soaps can be replaced with a good quality bar of soap. It should contain only sodium hydroxide and the oil of choice, optimally coconut oil or olive oil, and some other natural additives if desired, such as goat's milk.
- Shampoo and conditioner can be replaced with ghassoul clay or specific hair-centered soap (I love the clay, though!), and apple cider vinegar as a rinse afterwards. These work amazingly well and you should definitely try them.
- When your diet is on point, toothpaste really becomes a non-issue and, in most cases, you can just use a plain toothbrush with some water or dissolved sodium bicarbonate. It's best to use a very soft toothbrush so as not to attack the enamel. There are also toothpastes out

there incorporating calcium hydroxyapatite, which is a natural way to remineralize your teeth.

- **Perfumes:** You can find good quality organic ones or just make your own from essential oils.
- **Cleaning products:** At the very least, ventilate the room, use gloves and try natural alternatives to popular cleaning products, such as vinegar, sodium carbonate, Borax, etc.
- **Deodorant:** Use a natural oil-based product. They usually come in a small jar similar to skin cream. Diluted baking soda in water, about 1 tsp in 60 ml, works pretty well too. You can find a recipe on page 237.
- **Tap water:** For your municipal water supply, it makes total sense to get water filters. You can get a whole-house solution, which has the added benefit of cleaner water everywhere in your home, or you can get separate water filters for your different water outlets. This is not an ideal solution because charcoal works less efficiently at higher temperatures, so filtering it upstream before heating is preferable. There are water filters for the kitchen and the shower, which you can also use when taking a bath, with the mentioned caveat on the effectiveness of hot water filtration. A couple of little-known facts: When taking a hot shower, you absorb as many toxins from the water as you would in one week of drinking it. The pores open up and you absorb everything much more rapidly than you do with a cold shower. This is why when travelling I try to limit hot shower time to a minimum or even do cold showers only. When you live in a country with highly chlorinated water supplies, such as the US, also ventilate your bathroom regularly, since even the chlorinated water standing in the toilet will evaporate chlorine into the air, which you then in turn breathe in. Even if you don't have a filter, it's probably a good idea not to lie in your bathtub

while you let the water flow in. Instead, make it a little hotter, open a window and wait for a bit so at least some of the chlorine can evaporate into the air while you are ventilating. Minimizing chlorine intake by filtering your water at home will give your thyroid a much-needed break as well since chlorine displaces iodine, which our thyroid needs to make thyroid hormone. Read more about the significance of thyroid function for PKD in the section on hormone imbalance on page 197.

- **Medications:** It goes without saying that for all medications that you currently use it would probably be a good idea to find natural alternatives. These often work as well or better than drugs for the following simple reasons. Chemicals that pharmaceutical companies research are often derived from naturally occurring molecules, whose effects have been known for centuries. Pharmaceutical companies then make derivatives of these molecules, which are different enough for them to claim that they invented them, which in turn makes them able to file for a patent. That way they can make their money back, and much more in the following 20 years the patent lasts. This doesn't mean that these derivatives work better than the original molecules found in Nature; it just means these are the ones they're going to pour money into researching. These new molecules are of course foreign to our bodies and can have unintended consequences and side effects. Natural molecules, especially ones used for medicinal purposes for a long time, are known to our bodies and therefore will be much better tolerated in most cases.

Mitochondrial ROS (radical/reactive oxygen species)

As we have discussed before, damaged mitochondria in PKD have lost their ability to produce energy using respiration, so they cannot use oxygen for this process. However, they still consume oxygen, which for a long time had researchers confused. What are these damaged cells doing with the oxygen they are consuming? The answer: they produce free radicals. ROS, more specifically, is released by damaged mitochondria, which is then free to damage surrounding mitochondria and cells, contributing to a 'domino-effect'.

It is therefore vital for prevention of new cyst growth to scavenge these free radicals as soon as they are produced, and as close to the source as possible – which is inside the mitochondria. Specific supplements for this purpose exist and more are under development. The most affordable and sustainable way for sure is hydrogen gas dissolved in water, also called 'molecular hydrogen'. Produced using a hydrogen water generator or hydrogen tablets, this is a potent antioxidant highly specific to tissues that actually are under oxidative stress – very different and much deeper-penetrating than standard antioxidants such as vitamin C, which has a much broader and more non-specific effect. Hydrogen-water-producing bottles are widely available these days and are a great way to get a couple of daily doses of molecular hydrogen. In looking for a quality device, you want a high ppm reading, meaning a high concentration of molecular hydrogen. Therapeutic effects start around 1-3 ppm, but higher values are possible. Hydrogen tablets produce levels around 8 ppm. It makes sense to drink about 500 ml as quickly as possible to reach high peak concentrations in the body. Make sure to use clean, cold, filtered water only. Some other more specific mitochondrial ROS-targeting supplements include 'MitoQ' and a peptide called 'SS-31'.

Some other more specific mitochondrial ROS-targeting supplements include 'MitoQ' and a peptide called 'SS-31'.

Spike protein

Once an obscure topic, spike protein exposure today deserves special mention because of its newfound ubiquity. The spike protein, originally found on the surface of enveloped viruses like coronaviruses, has unique abilities to cause injury to, and even fuse together, cells[36] and to damage mitochondria, interfering with their ability to produce energy.[37]

There are three potential sources of spike protein to consider:

- Infection.
- Production inside the body in people who received a Covid-19 mRNA or DNA vaccine.
- Shedding from vaccinated people through air and bodily fluids. (Highest right after injection, likely declining over time.)

Concerns over shedding might surprise some readers, but these were initially raised after the Pfizer 2020 clinical protocol document advised study investigators to report skin contact or even contact through air inhalation between vaccinated people and pregnant women.[38, 39] Anecdotal reports and my personal experience align with these concerns raised by BioNTech and Pfizer.

Now, the body is quite adept at degrading natural spike protein that has been evolving and circulating in the community for millennia. It is a very different story to degrade a synthetic spike protein. To quote Dr Peter McCullough, MD: 'The human body does not seem to have enzymes that can break down this protein like it could any other natural protein and have us get rid of it. […] It's because this protein is not natural […]'

If you suspect you have been exposed to the virus or shedding recently, it makes sense to do a course of Base Spike Detox as outlined below alongside some immune system enhancement. High-dose vitamin D around 10 times the normal dose for a couple of days can boost the immune system to a great extent.

If you have received the Covid-19 vaccine, the considerations change, as this introduces mRNA or DNA into the body that turns many cells into spike-protein-producing factories. Contrary to popular belief, the mRNA that is present in most Covid-19 vaccines does not readily degrade. This is because of a change in its structure. Specifically, the insertion of pseudo-uridine was employed as a stability enhancer, an unprecedented move in human interventions, making it unclear how long it will persist in the body. One study analyzed the presence of the spike-protein coding mRNA for up to 60 days after the injection, which is when the study was terminated. At the end of the study, the mRNA was still present.[40]As long as the mRNA is present, the body will likely also continuously produce new spike protein, which means anyone affected would need to continuously do a spike-protein degrading therapy regimen to mitigate the potential damage. The insertion of pseudo-uridine didn't stabilize the mRNA without a cost, though: it makes it extremely prone to reading errors called 'frameshifting', which in addition to spike protein leads to the production of randomly assembled 'Frankenstein' proteins whose effects have not been studied.[41]

A simple starting point for a supplement regimen that degrades spike-protein and hopefully also 'Frankenstein' proteins, is the Base Spike Protein Detox published in a paper by Hulscher and colleagues in late 2023:[42]

- Nattokinase 2000 FU (100 mg) twice a day
- Bromelain 500 mg daily
- Nano-curcumin 500 mg twice a day.

You can find brand recommendations on my website, ReversingPKD.com/resources.

Now, keep in mind that nattokinase and bromelain also have blood-thinning effects, which might require you to adjust the dosage of any blood-thinning medication. On the other hand of course, spike protein increases the risk for clotting.[43]

This can also help with low white blood cell counts and a

suppressed immune system if these issues arose after receiving the Covid-19 mRNA or DNA vaccine.[44]

Ionizing radiation/X-rays

Whenever you are on a flight, you are exposed to radiation, which in turn leads to high oxidative stress. For example, a return transatlantic flight gives you about as much radiation as five chest X-rays. That's not a small dose, but it is spread out over a longer period, which might work in your favor. The most important thing is to do everything in your power to stay in ketosis during air travel. Ketones radically reduce radiation damage by quenching oxidative stress and upregulating the protective enzyme FOXO3, so this is a no-brainer… and it's free. Airline food is the worst anyway.

If you have to eat, make your meals keto. You can pack enough food to get you through your flight without consuming the usual terrible airline meals. Now if you decide to eat on the plane, I would recommend doing it in the proper circadian rhythm of your destination, so just adhere to the intermittent fasting schedule according to your destination. When you are eating, either on the plane or after landing, you can also add a couple of supplements to enhance your antioxidant defense and mitigate the effects of radiation:
- S-acetyl-glutathione or N-acetylcysteine
- Selenium
- Vitamin D
- Ubiquinol
- Vitamin C
- Alpha-lipoic acid.

Remember, antioxidant supplements tend to break a fast, so choose wisely. I personally remain in a fasted state during the flight to really ramp up the ketones and take the supplements shortly after landing.

All of this goes for having an X-ray or CT scan as well. Always advocate for an MRI instead, if you can. These are much gentler on the body and don't produce any X-rays. You can use PKD as a reason to give your doctor to avoid a CT scan. Of course, make very sure if you really need to have contrast fluid injected. I have had many scans in my life and I have never had contrast for them. In most cases, you can just refuse and they will still be able to tell you enough from the scan. The contrast itself is radioactive and poisonous. Should you have to take it, refer back to the supplement protocol above.

Non-ionizing radiation/EMFs

Have you been told that the radiation from your phone, your Wi-Fi router, your laptop, your smartwatch, etc, is nothing to be worried about? Well, think again. This outdated statement is based wholly on the assumption that radiation can only ever induce damage when it heats up biological tissue. While this is certainly dangerous – just think about sticking your hand into a microwave – this is far from being the only way that radiation can damage cells. So far in fact, that Robert F. Kennedy and his Children's Health Defense organization recently won a lawsuit against the FCC (Federal Communications Commission) in the US, showing that they had failed to update their guidelines on the safety of electromagnetic radiation for over 30 years. In this time, the FCC had ignored over 1000 new papers that had come out since the previous revision of their guidelines, showing conclusively that harm is being done by our everyday wireless devices. The FCC now has to rework its guidelines.[45]

So how does non-ionizing radiation cause harm? The summary is this:

> Outside of your cells there is a lot more calcium than inside of your cells, by a factor of about 20,000 to 100,000. This calcium obviously doesn't flow freely into and out of our cells

but is tightly regulated by voltage-gated calcium channels, also called VGCCs, in our cell membranes. Whenever intracellular calcium is increased, through a cascade of reactions, there is an increase in oxidative stress. This, in turn, can damage cell membranes, mitochondria, stem cells, and also DNA. This is exactly the type of injury we are trying to prevent.

Now, when we are exposed to non-ionizing radiation – for example, by being near a cell-phone transmitter tower, Wi-Fi router, or (even worse) using a Wi-Fi-connected laptop or just having a phone in our pockets that is not in airplane mode – these VGCCs can sense the radiation and they will mistake it for the signal to open the gate for calcium to flow into the cell. In one study, this process started after about 5 seconds.[46] So basically, your wireless devices are giving you inflammation exactly where you don't want it, inside your cells. If you are taking a calcium channel blocker for your blood pressure, you might be more protected from this. Mind you, they have other downsides though. For more information on the side effects of calcium channel blockers, refer to page 191.

There's a whole book on this topic by Dr Joseph Mercola called *EMF*d* and I highly recommend you read it if you want to know more about how this works.[47]

EMF mitigation strategies include:

- Convert your home to wired networking.
- Switch on Wi-Fi only as needed or at least use the timer function in your router.
- Switch your phone into airplane mode whenever you don't actively use it. When you're not using the internet, put it into airplane mode.
- When you're calling someone, use speakerphone and hold the phone away from your head while it's establishing a connection. This is when radiation is at its highest.
- Put your laptop in airplane mode; it is emitting radiation even when you're not connected to a Wi-Fi network.
- Don't use a microwave.

- Don't use an induction oven. They are great to save energy, but they emit high magnetic fields, which are easily measured with a trifield meter at home.
- Get an EMF-shielded tent or sleeping bag, or cover your walls with shielding paint.
- If you are working in a high-EMF environment, get an EMF-blocking T-shirt to cover your kidneys.
- Take antioxidants with your meals.
- Take ample amounts of magnesium, a natural calcium-channel blocker: around 1000 mg per day, divided into two to three doses is a good starting point.
- Get an EMF meter, such as the Acousticom 2, and make sure your sleeping quarters are in the green zone of radiation intensity.

Our bodies can usually cope with quite a high amount of stress, but it is cumulative. Some stress during the day and proper rest at night equals a stronger body. Non-stop stress equals burnout and breakdown. That's why you should pay the most attention to your bedroom when it comes to the mitigation of non-ionizing radiation. Give your body the chance to recover overnight and it will be much better equipped to handle a bit of radiation during the day. Funnily enough, PKD usually leads to a smaller amount of calcium inside the cells than normal, but there hasn't yet been any research showing a positive effect in this regard.

More supplements

For basic health

There are several supplements that most people need in the modern world. We tend to get way too little sunshine, minerals, omega-3 fatty acids, etc. So it is wise for most people to take somewhere in the ballpark of these doses of the following supplements daily, with or without PKD. Take into account if you might need food for absorption or if you want to activate or inhibit mTOR. Inhibition is for the fasting window, activation for feeding. If in doubt, or you forgot anything, you can still take it in the eating window.

In your eating window:
- Zinc: 15 mg
  Form: monomethionine, citrate, gluconate, glyinate
- Copper: 1 mg
  Form: bisglycinate, gluconate
- Iodine: 150-1000 mcg
  Form: kelp powder from clean sources
- Selenium: 200 mcg
  Form: selenomethionine
- Omega-3 fatty acids: 2000-3000 mg total EPA+DHA
  Form: fish oil, krill oil, algae oil
- Collagen: 15-20 g
  Form: Grass-fed collagen peptides
- Niacinamide: 50 mg at lunch and dinner
  Form: pure niacinamide powder.

In your fasting window:
- Vitamin D: 1000 IU per every 25 lb (11 kg) body weight
  Form: Vitamin D3
- Vitamin K2: 200 mcg
  Form: MK7
- Vitamin A: 10,000 IU
  Form: pre-formed retinol
- Magnesium: 500-1000 mg
  Form: citrate (high pH increase), malate (medium pH increase)
- Niacinamide: 50 mg mornings
  Form: pure niacinamide powder.

For longevity

NAD+ (nicotinamide adenine dinucleotide)

NAD+ is a coenzyme that is key to our metabolism. We have already mentioned it in the context of cyst growth, where cysts in the pathogenic mode of fermentation grow in an uncontrolled manner (page 6). Looking at this, one could assume that it is best to limit NAD+ wherever possible. However, this couldn't be further from the truth as it is a vital coenzyme for all of our cells that is essential, especially for mitochondrial health. It is involved extensively in DNA repair, inflammation control and immune system regulation. All of these are very relevant to PKD patients. DNA repair is crucial in preventing new cyst formation and inflammation control is vital in managing already existing cysts and pain.

NAD+ levels naturally become depleted with age, which negatively impacts our cellular health. Chronic inflammation as seen in PKD can deplete levels even further throughout the body. Maintaining youthful NAD+ levels throughout life is a good strategy to keep the body healthy as long as possible. There are expensive supplements on the market that claim to increase NAD+ levels, and they do seem to work to some extent, but there is a much more affordable and effective solution available, and it's a very cheap form of vitamin B3 called niacinamide, as you might've already gleaned from the list above.

Niacinamide acts as a precursor for NAD+ and is therefore very effective in replenishing NAD+ levels. The fact that nobody is marketing this is likely simply due to its very affordable nature. Since it is water-soluble, it doesn't last long in the body so it needs to be taken multiple times a day.

Since it also has an mTOR-inhibiting, autophagy-inducing effect, it can be taken morning, noon and evening and therefore serve as a continuous replenishment of NAD+. It also works synergistically with methylene blue (page 152) to facilitate energy production inside the mitochondria. The human equivalent dose for the dosage used in a recent mouse study would be about 2.5 mg per kilogram of body weight per day, divided into three doses.[48] So roughly 50-60 mg three times a day for the average person. If you buy powder in bulk and have a very small measuring spoon, you can keep this up for a very low price. You can look for a set of small measuring spoons that go down to a size as small as 1/64th of a teaspoon, which is the appropriate size for roughly 50 mg of niacinamide.

Glycine and collagen

Glycine is an amino acid, which means it is one of the building blocks of different proteins. It is part of what are called the 'conditionally essential' amino acids, meaning we can produce these ourselves, but not in a sufficient quantity. Therefore, we need to get glycine from food. So far, so good. However, glycine is dominant only in those foods that have fallen out of favor in the last couple of decades. These are foods that contain collagenous tissues like bone and skin, the most common being bone broth or the cartilage at the sides of your ribeye steak (that you usually leave on the plate).

What are the benefits of glycine?

Glycine is another mTOR inhibitor, promoting autophagy, and it reduces something known as AGEs (advanced glycation end products), which are basically caramelized proteins that accumulate in our bodies and which are very hard to get rid of. Searing meat and cooking at high temperatures both form AGEs. You can sometimes even see them as dark skin discolorations in elderly people. But just as the skin looks on the outside, the arteries look on the inside, so it's a worthwhile goal to limit AGEs.

Glycine also improves sleep quality through its calming effect on the brain, is a precursor to the master antioxidant glutathione and improves mitochondrial function,[49] especially when combined with N-acetylcysteine (NAC). It also offsets the aging effects of higher protein intakes from muscle meat.

Knowing all these benefits of glycine, straight up supplementation seems like a good idea. Studies have found that our bodies are in a substantial 10 to 15 gram glycine deficit every day.[50]

Other ways to get glycine are drinking or cooking with bone broth, eating grass-fed gelatin, or powdered grass-fed collagen peptides. Getting some of your glycine from collagen can have extra benefits. Collagen doesn't just include all the building blocks for connective tissue in our bodies, including the kidneys, but it's also a peptide, meaning it acts as a messenger molecule telling our bodies to form more collagen. Most likely because of this function, it can actually improve the integrity of the intestinal lining and enhance the function of tight junctions,[51] which are impaired through the PKD mutation.

Combining these insights, one could choose to supplement with 15 grams of grass-fed collagen and 10 grams of glycine per day, resulting in a total of 15 grams of glycine. Ideally this should be at the end of the daily eating window, when the body is preparing for the next fasting period, aiding sleep and recovery, but not disturbing the fasting window with too many amino acids.

For pain management

CBD oil

While the effectiveness of pain medication can be very individual, the use of CBD oil has surfaced as an effective and very safe intervention for kidney and liver pain. It is excreted through the stool and, if used in a sublingual preparation, preferably including DMSO, its effects can be felt within about 15 minutes.

A study of kidney transplant patients found that CBD oil was effective in reducing pain.[52] The study participants reported that they experienced a significant reduction in pain intensity and frequency after taking CBD oil. The study also found that CBD oil was safe and well-tolerated.

For regulating blood pressure

Minerals

Everybody knows that high blood pressure is a big no-no in PKD. And yes, this one the doctors got right. Higher blood pressure is correlated with faster disease progression and a higher rate of kidney cell injury. However, not everyone with PKD has high blood pressure. Not even in late stages. Isn't that interesting?

This means there are definitely lifestyle factors that can influence blood pressure in PKD, and they are mostly the same factors that can influence it in the general population. What are some of the requirements for healthy blood pressure? One of them is healthy mineral balance.

There is a common myth that table-salt (sodium chloride) intake will actually increase blood pressure. While that is the case for some people, it's not true for everybody. Why is that? These so-called salt-sensitive people are actually often times potassium deficient. You see, the body needs a proper balance between potassium and sodium to maintain healthy blood pressure. In our modern world, people don't get enough potassium from processed food so they become potassium deficient. Add to that a high amount of sodium in those same processed foods, and you got yourself a severe imbalance.

If you find that your blood pressure spikes after consuming salt, you are most likely deficient in potassium. Following the PKDproof program, you'll consume adequate amounts of potassium from natural sources like vegetables and grass-fed meats. These foods also still usually contain adequate calcium.

Of course, if your blood potassium levels are already very elevated, this changes the dynamic and you need to design your diet around lower potassium foods and potassium blockers, preferably with your doctor or a qualified practitioner.

Potassium is actually one of the few minerals that is still abundant in our current-day foods, because it is added into the soil via fertilizer. Most trace minerals have vanished from our soils over the last couple of hundred years, which is really no surprise when you think about it. Neither plants nor animals can actually make minerals. They just concentrate whatever they find in the soil. Back in the day, when humans ate food, they did not take its nutrients out of the food chain since they deposited their manure back into the earth, where the minerals it contained could then be redistributed and fed back to the plants, which would then feed them back to the animals and humans, completing a beautiful cycle.

With the industrialization of food and food processing, minerals are being sucked from the soil and then shipped away, sometimes to the other side of the planet, only for them to be eaten and then end up in some water-processing plant. Water processing companies try to redistribute the remnants from there but this system is far from perfect. As a result, humans have to add back minerals into the soil on a consistent basis for the plants to grow. However, not all minerals are needed by the plants to grow, and efficient as humans are, they are only adding back in through fertilizers the minerals that plants absolutely need to grow. Basically, all minerals and trace minerals except the ones that are being put back in with synthetic fertilizer or by holistic farming methods have been severely depleted. Think calcium, phosphorus, iron, zinc, magnesium… many of those essential minerals that used to be in our food are not there anymore in any appreciable amounts, so we don't get nearly enough of them. One 2004 study found 'reliable declines' in all minerals tested.[53]

This is the reason why I recommend everybody should take high doses of magnesium supplements. As noted at various times in this book, 500-1000 mg of elemental magnesium per day is a good start. This is actually very beneficial for blood pressure and essential for hundreds of bodily processes. If you get nighttime cramps, look at magnesium and sodium deficiency. Take some extra and see if it helps.

Many mammals actually have the capability to sense precisely the amounts of minerals that they need to take in for optimal bodily function. This is one of the reasons we have taste buds. If you have had enough of something, it doesn't taste that good anymore. You know this from many natural foods. As long as you don't process them to become hyperpalatable (super-tasty), your body knows when to stop. Or have you ever not been able to stop eating apples? One is nice, two is probably still fine, but after that you're not going to want to eat more of them.

While animals have honed this ability to detect what they need, what is still left of it in humans at least works quite well for gauging adequate salt intake. Since you will be eating an abundance of non-starchy vegetables and a healthy amount of meat, which both are an excellent source of potassium, you will have to balance that out by adding more sodium. When you get your salt from natural foods and just what you add yourself, your sense of taste will tell you exactly how much you need to eat. As long as you like the taste, add more.

Let me make this very clear: you don't need to restrict salt; you need to have adequate potassium intake from unprocessed, natural foods, thereby increasing your potassium to sodium ratio. This has the same effect as salt restriction but without running the risk of deficiencies.

Only if your blood potassium is too high does this template change. When your kidneys are not able to excrete potassium at the normal rate, it makes sense to go by your blood sodium, chloride and potassium values to gauge your individual optimal intake of potassium from vegetables and extra sodium from salt. To do this, work with your doctor or a qualified health coach or practitioner and titrate exactly how much you need.

Omega-3 supplements: The omega-6 to omega-3 ratio

A low omega-6 to omega-3 ratio, as we discussed in Chapter 4, at about 4:1 to 1:1 is optimal for physical functioning, is evolutionarily consistent and of course – you guessed it – correlates with lower blood pressure. The usual consumer of the 'standard American diet' (SAD) needs to take several grams of combined EPA+DHA per day to get there. If you keep to the diet recommendations in this book, you can probably get away with 2-3 grams of supplementary omega-3 per day. The only way to know where you stand is to get your own omega-6 to omega-3 index measured at your next doctor's appointment. You will probably have to pay for this yourself, but it is well worth it. There are even some online providers that will send you a finger prick test kit for convenient at-home measuring.

Colloidal silver

This one is a bit controversial in the conventional medical world. Silver has been used for hundreds of years for its antibacterial, antifungal and antiviral properties. People even used to put a pure silver coin into their milk bottles to make their milk keep for longer.

There is also a supplement form of silver that exhibits the same properties in the human body. Just be aware that the pharmaceutical industry is not interested in any of this and you will find many smear campaigns out there to try to discredit the use of colloidal silver. There are some scary stories of people turning blue after taking silver for many years. There actually are cases of this, but these individuals were not taking the proper form and in way too high a concentration, so deposition in the skin was possible. Amazingly this didn't result in any health issues, just a weird look, which goes to show how safe silver actually is. That being said, no ill effects have been reported with using a safe and low-concentration form of colloidal silver, such as 10 ppm silver hydrosol.

After hearing about this from a friend online, I have personally witnessed a severe drop in blood pressure of up to 20 points systolic about half an hour to an hour after ingesting 1 teaspoon of 10 PPM colloidal silver. The effect is repeatable and seems to last longer with every administration. If you look it up, you will find others reporting the same type of effects. While this is a completely unknown mechanism, the fact that not every PKD patient experiences high blood pressure opens up the possibility that this phenomenon is actually caused by something completely different, such as a cytomegalovirus infection, for example. Even a UTI can cause high blood pressure. So it's definitely possible that an antiviral, antibacterial solution like colloidal silver would have an effect against some of these pathogens, which would also explain why the effects seem to last longer with each administration. I'm not saying this has to be the mechanism or that it even works for everybody, but it's safe enough that anyone with high blood pressure should probably try this out for themselves. Of course, always adhere to the manufacturer's guidance on proper use and consult with a qualified practitioner if you are not sure what you're doing.

Melatonin

By now you are probably well aware of the great potential of melatonin to improve your sleep quality, since it is the main hormone for sleep. However, there is also good research showing that increasing melatonin levels at night reduces blood pressure in humans[54, 55] and good levels promote autophagy.[56] Getting a good night's sleep just became that much more important to your intermittent fasting regimen.

Melatonin alone might not be enough to get you off blood pressure meds, but it's certainly a great addition to the other natural methods we've talked about. About 2.5 mg orally one hour before sleep has been tested, and worked to reduce systolic and diastolic blood pressure by 6 and 4 mm Hg respectively – not bad for something that actually only has positive side effects. If you're using a sublingual spray, you can probably get away with an even smaller dosage, but the great thing is you can test this out for yourself. There are smart watches that can give you those readings even without waking you up, but getting the usual 24-hour blood pressure cuff test at your doctor's office will also suffice. My recommendation is to start off with the strategies in Chapter 9 on optimizing sleep and see how that influences your blood pressure, especially at night. You'll also find dosage recommendations there (page 109).

It's worth noting that the improvements were seen mostly in people whose blood pressure doesn't naturally decrease at night, which leads me to the suspicion that these people already had low melatonin production and might benefit most by incorporating the strategies to optimize sleep first. One study suggests that these improvements might take up to three weeks to occur so it might make sense to get a 24-hour blood pressure test one month after beginning to optimize your melatonin.[57]

Nattokinase

Nattokinase has gained recognition as a promising supplement in managing blood pressure. In a study conducted in 2008, this enzyme, derived from the Japanese food natto, was studied in a group of individuals aged between 20 and 80 years old.[58] Over eight weeks, the study participants received a daily dosage of one capsule of nattokinase containing 2000 FU (fibrinolytic units).

They experienced a noticeable reduction in blood pressure levels, with a net change in systolic and diastolic blood pressure of -5.55 mm Hg and -2.84 mm Hg respectively, compared with those on placebo. In addition, nattokinase is a great tool when it comes to mitigating blood clots, which are also an issue that is on the rise. If you have already had a blood clot or you suspect you have had one in the past, this should probably be in your supplement regimen. This works because nattokinase is a blood thinner, so if you are taking blood thinning medication, adjust accordingly. For many people, doses multiple times higher than the ones in the study can be safe and effective, so do your own research and double check with your doctor or qualified health practitioner.

Chapter 12

Common pitfalls

'Keto flu'

One of the first hurdles you may encounter when switching to keto is the infamous 'keto flu'. Some get it, some don't. This is not a real influenza but a collection of symptoms that can occur as your body adjusts to burning fat for energy. These symptoms can include fatigue, headaches, nausea, dizziness, irritability and muscle cramps. Typically, keto flu symptoms will last for a few days to a week, but hydration and electrolyte balance can significantly help mitigate them. Your need for salt increases by a factor of up to four times when in ketosis, and the symptoms of sodium deficiency are mostly identical with the symptoms of 'keto flu'. Make sure, therefore, to salt your food to taste, supplement with ample magnesium, drink enough water so your urine looks slightly yellow and, most importantly, eat your organic veggies and grass-fed beef as they contain lots of electrolytes as well.

Electrolyte imbalance

When you switch to keto-burning, your kidneys will begin to excrete more water and electrolytes like sodium, potassium and magnesium. This imbalance can exacerbate the symptoms of keto flu and cause additional problems like muscle cramps and arrhythmias. Just as with keto flu, pay attention to magnesium, salt and adequate food intake.

Low ketone readings

If you are struggling to hit your desired target ketone levels (see page 114), there are a couple things to keep in mind. If you just started out and you are not getting into ketosis yet, don't despair. It can take a week or two to get into ketosis, depending on your degree of metabolic flexibility. Now, if you are past this period and ketones are still on the low side, take another look at your macronutrient intake. Carbohydrates should be below 40 g per day, your protein should be around 0.6 g per pound of body weight, and the rest of your macros should be fat. If you're already doing this and you are still not reaching your desired level of blood ketones, you can modify your macros more.

If you have been on a ketogenic-style diet for a long time and you have seen higher ketones in the past than you are seeing now, this is actually an expected change, as you are getting fat-adapted. The longer you are on a ketogenic diet, the more efficient your body becomes at using fat for energy directly and will use a large part of dietary fats for energy production before even converting it to ketones, the degree of which might be dependent on your genetics. A 2017 rat study actually described this phenomenon. Rats were fed a ketogenic diet for eight months, and while their blood BHB levels were 1.25 mM on average in the beginning, on the same diet they had dropped to as low as 0.66 mM at the end of the study.[1] That's half as many ketones after fat adaptation. This might be because, in a fat-adapted person, really the only part of the body that can't use fatty acids directly is the brain, as fats cannot penetrate the blood-brain barrier, but ketones can. The rest of the body is so adapted, that it can happily use fatty acids for energy directly.

Whether this adaptation has an impact on the amount of

cyst growth in ketogenic dieting for PKD is not known at this stage. Maybe it's all about switching your body to an alternative fuel source, away from cyst-feeding glucose. But maybe the additional medicinal properties that ketones have also play a role. It's best to judge by your own results for now.

So let's assume you still want to increase your blood ketone levels, maybe because you aren't seeing results yet. You can 'force' your body to produce more ketones by lowering your protein and increasing your fat intake even more. We are approaching unnatural territory here so this might be difficult to sustain long-term. You may want to try reaching a ratio of fat to protein-and-carbs of 1.5:1 up to 4:1, meaning 1.5 times or even four times as many grams of fat as grams of protein and carbs combined, with 2:1 being used in some of the ketogenic trials on cancer.[2] Now, depending on your appetite, this might lead you to lowering protein below your minimum requirements so this is definitely a judgment call and should at most be an intermittent regimen, possibly combined with glutamine inhibition, that you interrupt with periods of ample protein intake, as it is vital for muscle mass and kidney regeneration. It's much more sustainable to keep your minimum protein intake and add on extra fats, increasing total calorie intake.

As mentioned on page 60, the reason this works is that your body can only metabolize fatty acids directly when it has enough oxaloacetate, which is needed as a catalyst for the reaction. Oxaloacetate is provided through protein and carbohydrate intake. So, when your ratio of fat to protein-and-carbohydrate rises beyond a certain point, you deplete your oxaloacetate reserves and force your body to convert a larger part of the fat to ketones.

Another hack to lower blood glucose and raise ketone levels is to keep your meals to 300 kcal each and space them out evenly over the day. This can also be combined with a slight 20% calorie deficit for even better results. Of course, this can only be sustained for as long as you are in the healthy BMI range.

It also makes sense to monitor your blood glucose after meals so you can gauge your individual reaction to specific foods with regards to blood glucose and ketones. Sometimes unknown food sensitivities can raise your cortisol levels, and thereby your blood glucose, which in turn inhibits ketogenesis.

Bad breath

Some people notice a metallic or fruity smell on their breath when they first go into ketosis. This is due to the production of a type of ketone called acetone, which can be released in the breath. The smell is usually temporary and diminishes as your body becomes more efficient at using ketones for energy.

Remembering to track your progress

As discussed in Chapter 10, Tracking your progress, it's essential to keep a close eye on various markers to ensure that your diet is working for you even though this may feel tedious at times. This involves not just tracking blood ketone levels but also paying attention to other parameters like blood pressure, second morning urine pH and food intake, as we discussed. Don't just assume everything's going to plan; make sure that it is. If it's not, adjust your approach until the values are in the desired optimal ranges. As the saying goes, you can't hack what you don't track. Only when you feel confident that you are able to predict the results based on your intuition and adherence to the regimen, you should begin lowering the frequency of testing until you can finally just check in every couple of weeks or even months to see if your feeling is still correct or if something has changed.

Hunger and meeting macros

With this way of eating, hunger should not be one of your issues. It is very important we adequately nourish the body to get it to an optimal state of healing. In the beginning you may find it difficult to hit your targets, so it is highly recommended to use the food tracking apps, such as Cronometer, as we discussed before. Make sure you are hitting your calorie and protein targets as calculated. Carbs will not play a major part most days of the week and fat will make up most of your remaining calories after accounting for protein. If you are concerned about excessive weight loss, simply eat more calories. Use homemade fat bombs (page 231) to boost your calorie intake if necessary. Some sample recipes have been included at the end of this book. More can also easily be found online. Just make sure you keep to the list of allowed ingredients.

Food cravings

Whenever you experience food cravings, ask yourself this simple question: Have I met my protein needs for today? If the answer is no, get more protein in. This is the most common driver of food cravings. The body will crave more food until protein needs are met. After you eat your protein, give yourself 15 minutes for satiety to set in. After this period, you can give yourself permission to make and eat whatever food you might be craving, if it is on the Bulletproof Diet, or make a substitute if it's not.

It's important you are aware of these substitutes, since switching your diet should never be about sacrificing flavor or satiety. This has to work for the long term. So where protein can't dispel the cravings, you can make a healthy substitute. You might be surprised at what replacements you can make for popular desserts and snack foods. Coconut flour is the preferred base for most of these, but you can also use macadamia flour or blanched-almond flour. We use blanched-almond flour because the husks have been removed, which contain most of the antinutrients and mold. However, even blanched almond flour might still be reasonably high in oxalic acid, which we are trying to limit where possible (page 45). Occasional use is okay, but if you're making something to be consumed regularly, go for macadamia or coconut flour.

You can also make keto-compatible ice cream that tastes phenomenal and is made up of mostly eggs, saturated fat and erythritol. In addition, you can find keto substitutes for many foods, even in supermarkets; just make sure you check the ingredients so that you are not consuming additional toxins. Staples for snacks include 85%, or darker, chocolate, beef jerky and raw organic macadamia nuts.

Concerns about too much protein

Even though we have addressed this topic before, the concern about 'too much protein' has been hammered home by most physicians so patients are understandably confused when they hear they should be consuming more protein than traditionally suggested. The old paradigm was based on the assumption that higher protein intake somehow worsened kidney function by 'stressing' the kidneys too much. However, this simplified view is not really supported by the science. It is true that if one's kidney function declines too much, all sorts of waste products, including remnants of protein metabolism, accumulate in the blood, but this is where most people make an error of judgment. Just because an accumulation of waste products and low kidney function occur at the same time doesn't mean that these waste products are the *cause* of lower kidney function. On the contrary, may I remind you that protein and its amino acids are essential building blocks to retain kidney function and repair cellular damage. Protein is needed as a necessary building block to repair and maintain healthy kidney tissue, as well as increase kidney function.

Now, when there is actually an elevated level of uremic toxins, such as blood urea nitrogen (BUN) in the blood, that is where some symptoms such as fatigue and loss of appetite can set in. Consequently, this is where adjustments are necessary (see Chapter 4 on the Bulletproof Diet template, and Chapter 6 on adjustments for low kidney function).

Chapter 13

About common medications and PKD

Statins

Very commonly, patients will get the recommendation to start on a statin drug because cholesterol levels are deemed high by their doctor. Statins are actually the most profitable drugs on the planet, bringing in just about $19 billion per year. So you can imagine that many doctors will be inclined to prescribe them if given the chance.

You can rest assured that cholesterol itself is not the problem and statins will not fix whatever problem there may be. Cholesterol is less like the fat that is clogging your sink, as is still a popular analogy, and more like the fire brigade rushing to the scene of the fire. Taking statins will only remove the firefighters, not prevent or put out the fire. The fire, which in this case is inflammation, is usually caused by diet, especially the aforementioned seed oils and processed foods.

Now, high cholesterol levels in themselves aren't actually an issue. They may just be a sign of a higher-than-average intake of saturated fat. The reference levels on most blood test panels were established in a population eating a diet low in saturated fat, hence these levels do not apply to people eating a well-designed ketogenic diet on most days. When cholesterol levels are high in people on a low-fat diet, that might be a cause for concern. In high-fat eaters this is just a natural, expected outcome.

Now there are parameters on a cholesterol blood panel that are more interesting – for example, we want to see triglycerides lower than HDL. This ratio correlates well to bodily inflammation and the lower the triglycerides, the lower the inflammation. The higher the HDL, the higher the intake of saturated fats.

Triglycerides < HDL

Another good parameter to check is the so-called 'remnant cholesterol'. You can calculate it easily by subtracting HDL and LDL from your total cholesterol.

Total cholesterol - LDL - HDL = Remnant cholesterol (RC)

You want this to be at least below 15 mg/dl, but ideally zero. Remnant cholesterol correlates with VLDL (very low density lipoprotein), which is much more expensive to get tested. Both RC and VLDL are significant risk factors for cardiovascular disease.

For an even more detailed assessment of your cholesterol results, you can use the free report calculator over at cholesterolcode.com. If you have trouble finding it, the up-to-date links are always on the resources page for this book at ReversingPKD.com/resources.

Blood pressure medicines

If you are reading this and you have high blood pressure, you might be asking yourself: 'What are the best medications to take, what are the pros and cons of each and how can I potentially reduce or eliminate my need for them?' While I'm not going to elaborate on all the available medications extensively, and you can read the list of side effects for yourself, I want to highlight some specific aspects of some of these medications that you might want to consider.

Calcium channel blockers

This group of medications includes amlodipine and verapamil, among others. They lower blood pressure by stopping calcium from entering heart and artery cells. Calcium is needed for those muscles to contract more strongly, so blocking its entry will lower the pumping force put out by these muscles in contraction. Rat studies have shown faster disease progression in rat models of PKD. One 2017 study on calcium channel blockers showed increased kidney weight and cyst index in a rat model of PKD.[1] Mechanistically this makes sense: the fact that calcium flow is already impaired in PKD opens up the possibility that this type of blood pressure medication could speed up disease progression in PKD in humans, just as it does in rats. Also in a 2015 study, the use of calcium channel blockers was linked to higher mortality rates compared to other blood-pressure-lowering medications.[2]

Beta-blockers

Beta-blockers like propranolol, nadolol, labetalol, etc. work by blocking beta-receptors throughout the body. Some beta-receptors are present on the heart, waiting for epinephrine (adrenaline) to attach to them and give the signal to increase heart rate and contraction force when pumping blood. When these receptors are blocked by the medication, the heart beats more slowly and with less force, lowering blood pressure.

However, these receptors don't just exist on the heart but throughout the body. One place that's particularly problematic is the pineal gland. Here, beta- and alpha-receptors are needed to regulate melatonin production, which means the production of our sleep hormone. Melatonin levels are already generally lower in people with high blood pressure and will be further reduced by beta-blockers by up to 80%.[2]

If you are taking beta-blockers and you don't intend to stop, one study suggests that taking extra melatonin at night can alleviate some of the sleep problems associated with these drugs.[3] The dosage used was 2.5 mg of melatonin before bed for three weeks. (Refer back to pages 107-109 and 177-178 for more on melatonin.)

RAS inhibitors

RAS-, or renin-angiotensin system, inhibitors are widely used to treat high blood pressure. These drugs work by blocking parts of the RAS, in effect inhibiting the narrowing of blood vessels. They include ACE inhibitors, ARBs and direct renin inhibitors. Studies in mice and humans reveal that these medications can lead to a significant thickening of the small arteries within the kidneys.[4] This thickening is due to the growth and change of so-called renin cells.

Renin cells, under the influence of RAS inhibitors, undergo a transformation. Instead of maintaining their usual function, they start to surround the vessel walls and cause the accumulation of muscle cells and other substances around the vessels. This leads to blockage in blood flow, localized lack of blood supply and scarring within the kidneys. Also, a 2023 study of over 30,000 patients found an 11% increased risk of stroke that required hospitalization.[5]

Now I don't know about you, but triggering unusual growth anywhere in the kidneys sounds like a potential issue for PKD patients to me, mechanistically speaking.

Another important point to note is that, while this is usually not permanent, since blood pressure inside the kidneys is also reduced by these medications, filtering capacity is lowered, resulting in a higher creatinine level and lower eGFR for the period of use. If your function is low, it may become necessary to stop taking these to recover some kidney function.

Tolvaptan

Tolvaptan emerged in 2015 by getting approval in the EU for treatment of ADPKD. It was first researched by Otsuka in 1998 and secured approval in 2010 for addressing low blood sodium levels. It works as a vasopressin receptor antagonist, as vasopressin is dysregulated in PKD. Clinical trials initially caused hope, with findings of up to 50% reduction in cyst growth. A recent pooled long-term study showed patients not using tolvaptan lost 16.4 points in GFR over a five-year period while patients using the drug lost 12.4 points.[6]

These results are attained in the context of the extreme thirst and need for urination that tolvaptan creates. Patients on this drug often consume up to 7 litres of water per day, which in itself has been hypothesized to be a likely reason for the benefits that were seen. The initial study has been criticized from the get-go for not having a placebo group with fluid intake similar to the treatment group. The consistent need for bathroom breaks can severely impact quality of life while only slightly slowing progression towards kidney failure.

In addition, the FDA has restricted their recommendations to a mere 30 days of use[7] and no use at all in people with underlying liver disease. Needless to say, most PKD patients also have cysts in their liver. The approach in most doctors' offices right now is to prescribe the medication anyway and wait for liver markers to deteriorate. Whenever this happens, the medications are usually stopped as this type of liver injury can be irreversible and sometimes fatal.

The enthusiasm around tolvaptan primarily stems from the pharmaceutical industry's inclination towards repurposing existing, approved drugs, a tactic favored to bypass the high costs and extensive logistics of developing new drugs.

Pain medication

NSAIDs

NSAIDs, which stands for 'non-steroidal anti-inflammatory drugs', work by inhibiting Cox-1 and Cox-2 enzymes, involved in regulating blood flow in the kidneys. Restricting the activity of these enzymes reduces kidney blood flow and oxygen delivery, potentially inducing direct damage and function loss. NSAIDs can also increase sodium and fluid retention.

In the context of PKD, utilizing NSAIDs is generally discouraged for chronic pain and long-term use. Acetaminophen/paracetamol is recommended by the PKD Foundation as a safer alternative, so let's look at that one next.

Acetaminophen/Paracetamol

Also called tylenol, this too is a cyclo-oxygenase (COX) pathway inhibitor. Acetaminophen appears to inhibit the COX enzyme in the central nervous system, but not in peripheral tissues, such as the kidneys. This is why it is not thought to have the same negative effects on the kidneys as NSAIDs.

This drug is metabolized in the liver, while NSAIDs are metabolized in the kidneys. This means that acetaminophen is less likely to build up in the kidneys and cause damage. Still, acetaminophen use was correlated with a faster progression towards kidney failure in a population study in the *New England Journal of Medicine*.[8] About 10% of people went into kidney failure due to their use of acetaminophen/paracetamol when compared with the low usage group. However, even the low usage group was allowed to take up to 104 pills of acetaminophen per year, so the drug could have led to even more cases of kidney failure that were not discovered due to this relatively high threshold.

While stomach bleeding and ulcers are mostly an issue in NSAIDs, acetaminophen/paracetamol can also lead to these same problems, albeit at a lower rate.

Aspirin

Aspirin has actually been touted as a good long-term daily medication to take, especially with increased age.

One study in 146,152 people aged over 60 actually concluded: 'Aspirin use 3 or more times per week was associated with reduced risk of all-cause cancer, gastrointestinal cancer, and colorectal cancer mortality.'[9] However, the potential downside of a long-term aspirin regimen like this is also related to one of its upsides, namely its blood-thinning effect, which, while preventing blood clots, also increases the risk for gastrointestinal bleeding and the potential rupturing of cholesterol plaques. So while it can prevent a heart attack by maintaining blood flow, the same anticoagulant effect can also lead to bleeding into cholesterol plaques,[10] potentially causing a heart attack.

Chapter 14

Barriers to healing:
Where to go from here

If the strategies in this book after a couple of months don't lead to the desired results or you are even progressing downhill, even though your pH, ketones, food intake, supplementation and sleep schedule are all in line, it may be time to go on the hunt for deeper issues. Even though I won't be able to go into detail on everything here, I want to give you some hints as to what could possibly be impeding your body's ability to heal.

Glutamine and glucose levels

If you are not seeing results yet, it's definitely possible that your individual biology requires higher ketone levels than you are currently seeing, or that your PKD is still having too much access to glutamine. It therefore makes sense to start off with increasing your ratio of fat to protein-and-carbohydrate to raise your blood ketones to 2-3 mmol/l (more on page 61), and possibly slightly restrict calories and meal sizes to lower your blood glucose to the therapeutic range of 55-65 mg/dl. This is also the time when you can begin to implement some glutamine blocking strategies for an increased effect (see page 152).

Hormone imbalance

A very common issue, not just in PKD patients but in the

population in general, is thyroid dysfunction. As I have said, the thyroid can be thought of as a sort of master thermostat of your body, and if it is not functioning optimally, healing can be a very difficult process. There is also a close interaction between thyroid and sex hormones, which makes it even more important to get both of them checked and corrected if necessary.

To learn more about how to best address thyroid issues, I recommend the book *The Paleo Thyroid Solution* by Elle Russ.[1] It goes into detail on how to treat yourself whenever a good doctor or endocrinologist just cannot be found, as is often the case.

Sex hormones should also be kept in balance, especially in menopause for women and in old age for men; they can decrease significantly, so it is important to work with a skilled practitioner who is well-versed in interpreting something like the DUTCH test, which stands for 'dried urine test for comprehensive hormones'. They will assess your current state and help you to correct any kind of hormone imbalance, which will go a long way to giving your body the energy that it needs to repair and rebuild.

Another hormone that will appear on the DUTCH test panel is cortisol. This is our primary stress hormone and after a period of chronic stress it can be severely depressed, causing, fittingly, depression. I personally faced this challenge and I have seen great success using the Kalish method developed by Dr Dan Kalish. (See also his book *The Kalish Method: Healing the Body, Mapping the Mind*[2]) He uses tightly titrated doses of hormone precursors to replenish just enough cortisol to match what your body used to make, which helps it to be able to regain its strength without being overdosed and stopping its own production. In my personal experience it took me about six months of supplementing with pregnenolone, which is a precursor to cortisol, to resolve my low cortisol. However, this is not the solution for everyone, since it doesn't always have to be production that is low; there can also be significant loss of cortisol by conversion to cortisone. In many cases, instead of increasing production, this conversion has to be inhibited with something like licorice extract. Let me stress again that it is very important a trained practitioner interprets your test results to give you an adequate dosage recommendation as there are many factors involved.

Low cortisol, which is also sometimes referred to as 'burnout' or 'adrenal fatigue', is usually caused by chronic stress, especially of the kind that cannot be resolved easily. A surefire way to get a human into low cortisol is to put them in an environment where they are constantly stressed, possibly afraid and have no means of recourse. No matter how well you correct it, in this kind of environment the issue will always resurface or might not even resolve. So if you are in a situation like that, find a way to escape it. Quit your job, cut ties with 'that person' if necessary, study something else, switch universities, move house, whatever is needed. Remove the stressor or you will find yourself in this situation again. Believe me, I speak from experience.

Heavy metal poisoning

Another big one can be heavy metal toxicity, as the kidneys filter waste products from the blood, including heavy metals, which in turn can injure the kidneys leading to cyst growth. Nowadays heavy metals lurk everywhere, but even though you will be avoiding common sources such as tuna on the Bulletproof Diet, you might still have a significant burden of toxic heavy metals. One way to find out if this is an issue is for you is to get a heavy metal challenge urine test. This is done by injecting DMPS, EDTA or a similar chelating agent and then measuring your urine 90 minutes later to see which heavy metals and how much of them can be found in it. The same injections can then later be used to pull more and more of these heavy metals out of your body.

However, this is still a controversial technique, as minerals and heavy metals are removed indiscriminately at the same time.

There is also limited evidence from animal models showing when DMPS is administered with an acute dose of mercury, this can lead to additional injury.[3] However, this is an extreme scenario most likely not applicable to everyday life in humans. In another case of induced mercury toxicity in mice, DMPS has even been shown to rescue the induced nephropathy.[4]

There are other ways of getting rid of heavy metals, such as taking niacin before an infrared sauna for something like the Andy Cutler protocol. If you're specifically dealing with mercury poisoning, a new substance called emeramide seems to be the best way to get rid of it for now, but it is not easy to obtain and is usually sold by Chinese manufacturers while the American version is still waiting for approval.

Should you have mercury amalgam fillings in your teeth, you should not begin on any detox program, as this will only pull out more of that mercury. Please find a biological dentist who is experienced in removing these fillings without causing even more toxicity in the process, which routinely wrecks patients when the procedure is performed by a standard dentist. An ecological dentist will use a rubber dam and sophisticated ventilation and advise on detox strategies afterwards. I repeat: do not begin any kind of mercury detox while amalgam fillings are still in place. This will increase the amount of mercury leaching from your fillings into your body and raise the risk of redistribution into sensitive tissues such as the brain. Once the fillings have been removed, your dentist can then also guide you through a mercury detox program.

There are several directories online to find a biological dentist in your area.

A very interesting way to get rid of heavy metals that is emerging in the holistic health field is mineral rebalancing. Pioneered by Dr Lawrence Wilson, it typically involves a hair mineral analysis test to measure the levels of various minerals in the body, identifying any deficiencies and imbalances that need addressing. This is important as it guides the dosage of minerals and nutrients to restore balance, allowing the body to naturally expel heavy metals. This is particularly important as heavy metals can replace essential minerals in the body, disrupting normal bodily functions. Mineral rebalancing creates an internal environment that helps the body to let go of heavy metals in a gentle way, as opposed to chelation therapy, which can potentially leave enzymes non-functioning due to abrupt metal removal without adequate minerals as a replacement. This is likely the best approach as it requires no IVs or chemicals and keeps any extra burden off the detox organs. To learn more, you can visit Dr Wilson's website at drlwilson.com and refer to the practitioner directory.

Mold toxicity and chronic infections

Many homes nowadays have mold issues and, while inhabitants often think nothing of it or use quick and dirty methods of trying to get rid of mold themselves, these attempts can result in the mold excreting even more spores as it responds to being threatened. This can make people in the house, especially those performing the removal, even more sick. To add to that, mold can even colonize the body, usually in the sinuses or the gut. If this happens, a more involved process of killing, and then removing, mold and its toxins has to be performed. It can be quite difficult to find any kind of doctor who is versed in this; a good start is looking for a practitioner trained in the Brewer protocol. You can find out if you have a mold issue with the mycotoxin tests offered by Real-Time labs or Great Plains laboratory (see ReversingPKD.com / resources).

One interesting tell-tale sign of mold toxicity are frequent shocks of static electricity when touching metal surfaces. In short, mold toxicity can lead to ADH (antidiuretic hormone) dysregulation, which in turn increases sweat production. This increases the likelihood of experiencing static shocks.

A good book recommendation to learn more about mold toxicity and other obscure toxicities is *Toxic* by Neil Nathan, MD.[5] It also goes into detail on chronic Lyme infections and lesser-known conditions such as mast cell activation syndrome (MCAS). Issues like chronic infections are often intertwined with mold- or heavy metal toxicity and it can take some time to find what's at the root of the problem in your specific case. Treating the chronic infection itself can often times prove futile, as the body is burdened with an underlying toxicity that prevents the immune system from completely resolving any chronic infection.

Root canals

This procedure might be among the worst things that you can possibly get done at any dentist's office. Dentistry is the only profession where a dead body part is actually left remaining inside the body. Altogether 4999 out of 5000 extracted teeth that received a root canal and were sent to a lab by Dr Huggins and Dr. Boyd Haley were actually found to be infected.[6] If you have a root canal, the chances are you are carrying around a chronic infection and are swallowing toxic bacteria... and their poisons, such as endotoxin. There is already one mechanism by which a root canal could make PKD a lot worse, but of course there are many others as well.

A root canal should be removed as soon as possible, and if replaced, should only be replaced by a pure ceramic implant with no metal parts, as those can leech metal into the body and cause disturbance in the electrical fields, as well as generate a micro-current inside the mouth. It makes sense to find a biological dentist to perform this procedure as mentioned above.

Nutrient deficiencies

Nutrient deficiencies can be an insidious way to keep your body from healing. While the PKDproof program will take care of some of these, you might need additional supplementation for some nutrients and others might take time to build back up from a severe deficiency. When you're not healing after several months of adhering to the diet regimen and meeting the target levels in home tracking, it might make sense to work with a practitioner to assess your individual health status. Some very common nutrient deficiencies include:

- Vitamin D
- Vitamin K2
- Zinc
- Copper
- Iodine
- Selenium
- Magnesium
- B-vitamins.

To address nutrient deficiencies, finding an orthomolecular medicine practitioner would be a good option. One comprehensive directory can be found at orthomolecular.org.

Getting help with barriers to healing

Now if you need help putting the strategies outlined in this book into practice, or you have already done it but just can't seem to get the results that you are looking for, you might want to schedule an appointment and see if I can help you find that breakthrough. I do still accept clients in my personal health coaching program specializing in reversing PKD; you can schedule a free short assessment call on www.ReversingPKD.com.

If you believe your health issues lie in a different area than

PKD, finding a practitioner who is versed in holistic methods of healing can be quite a challenge. Believe me, I've been there. While I won't suggest any specific practitioners to you in this book, I have achieved the most by finding out which devices or protocols really good practitioners talk about in the books, shows or blogs that I find about any particular topic and then getting in touch with manufacturers or the institutes teaching those protocols or selling those devices and asking them for a practitioner directory, or even personal recommendations for my area.

Using this method, I have found exceptional doctors from general practitioners to hormone specialists, dentists and beyond.

Conclusion

Congratulations! By finishing this book, you are now one of the most well-informed PKD patients on the planet. Just a couple of years ago none of these interventions were on the radar of scientists, much less doctors or patients. Some studies have been done every now and then over the past decades, but nobody had put two and two together and realized that a well-balanced intermittent ketogenic diet like the Bulletproof Diet and regular fasting periods could have such a profound impact on the progression of PKD.

When I started my Facebook group and began publicizing this information, nobody had heard of this approach and even I was only beginning to understand why it worked. Since, then, we have been so lucky that the scientific community has slowly woken up to this unbelievable opportunity to improve the lives of so many PKD patients, staving off or even preventing dialysis. Research papers on this diet for PKD patients specifically still do not exist, and studies on the effect of ketones in general on PKD patients are in their infancy. In general, scientific studies on dietary interventions are always hard to find funding for, as there is no financial incentive for pharmaceutical companies to sponsor this type of research.

This makes it so much more important for patients to connect, but it can become difficult in terms of social media, as pharmaceutical companies also increase their grip on patients' communities there. Shadow banning and censoring content that might decrease profits, such as this book, are a real concern. To combat any type of censorship in the future, I will always link the groups where patients can connect without censorship on different social media networks over on my website www.ReversingPKD.com under 'community'. Also, make sure to enter your email address if you want to stay in contact should one of these groups be shut down.

So please join our group on Facebook, MeWe, or whatever other networks will be available next. We need you all to share your progress so more people will see that this approach actually works. Is your GFR going up after a couple of months of implementing the strategies in this book? Is your kidney volume going down? Is pain decreasing? What about your BUN or uric acid levels?

Post about it on one of our groups or on your own profile on any of the platforms and tag @reversingpkd or use the hashtags #reversingpkd and #pkdproof.

I wish you all the best on your healing journey. You are now well-equipped to take on PKD and tip the proverbial scales in your favor with the diet, supplements and all the different strategies that make up the PKDproof program. Find what works for you, and then tell others about it. Other patients depend on you. Invite them to the group, forward them a link to buy this book, or give them a printout of the Quick Start guide (page 209).

The medical profession will probably remain oblivious to all of this for at least another 10 years, but you can help speed up this process as well. Talk to your doctor about this book or give them a copy. Your doctor works for you, so if they're not interested, it might be time to find someone else who will be your ally on this journey.

I will see you out there. All the best, and heal well!

Felix

Appendices

I. The Quick Start guide for reversing PKD

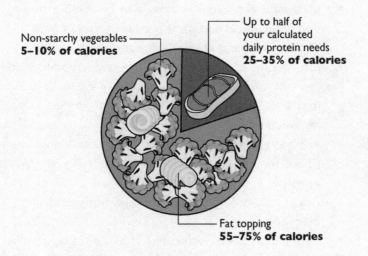

Non-starchy vegetables
5–10% of calories

Up to half of
your calculated
daily protein needs
25–35% of calories

Fat topping
55–75% of calories

The PKDproof plate

Dietary guidelines

- Adopt a **ketogenic diet** like the Bulletproof Diet 5-6 days
  a week with an emphasis on high-quality saturated fats,
  adequate protein and minimal carbohydrates.
- Main protein sources: Choose grass-fed beef or lamb as
  your primary meat. Sockeye salmon occasionally.

- Main fat sources: Grass-fed butter, ghee, organic coconut oil, tallow/beef dripping, avocado.
- Carbohydrate limit: Restrict your daily carbohydrate intake to less than 40 grams
- Protein intake: Calculate your protein needs based on your body weight. Aim for approximately 0.6 grams of protein per pound (0.45 kilos) of body weight.
- Calories: Consume adequate calories, especially if you already have a low body weight. Multiply your optimal body weight in pounds by 14 for a rough estimate.
- Macronutrients: Your calories will be coming from fat first, your calculated protein intake second and a maximum of 40 grams of vegetable-source carbohydrates.
- Incorporate a variety of non-starchy vegetables like broccoli, cauliflower, salads and leafy greens into your meals as the main bulk. Enjoy them alongside your grass-fed beef or lamb.
- Salt food to taste to balance sodium and potassium. Check for dietary potassium deficiency if you are salt sensitive.
- Add 1 tbsp of MCT (medium chain triglycerides) oil to every meal.
- Avoid most dairy, processed foods, alcohol, starches, seed oils, sugar, spinach and other very high oxalic acid foods (more than 100 milligrams (mg) per 100 grams (g))
- Adjust protein intake according to your GFR and BUN (blood urea nitrogen level), and adjust all food intake according to phosphorus and potassium blood levels.

Hydration

- Consume about **3 liters of water** daily to support kidney health and overall wellbeing. Slightly yellow urine is what we're shooting for.

Supplementation

- Start supplementation with **magnesium**. Aim for a daily intake of **4-6 mg per pound of body weight**.
- Add **vitamin D3** (1000 IU per every 25 lb per day) if you are in the sun less than an hour per day shirtless, and **vitamin K2 MK7**, 200 micrograms (mcg) per day
- If restricting protein, **make up for the difference with Ketoanalogs of essential amino acids**: 1 g KAEAAS = 2 g protein.

Fasting

- Implement a **16 to 18-hour intermittent fasting window** between dinner and breakfast 6 days a week to promote autophagy (see page 20) for cellular cleanup and repair.
- If you have average or low fitness, incorporate **a 36-72-hour modified protein fast** once a month.
  Breakfast: Butter and MCT coffee
  Lunch: 1 cup bone broth with 150 g Brussels sprouts for a 150-pound human.
- Optional: include glutamine blocking strategies in your 36-72 hour fast.

Carbohydrate refeed day

- Designate 1-2 days per week for a carbohydrate refeed.
- Options for carb refeed days include organic non-Chinese white rice, **avocado, or cucumber sushi with MCT oil and salt**, sweet potato, and **organic fruit**.
- If you want to enjoy a treat like gluten-free pizza, this is the day but remember to take activated charcoal with it to mitigate potential negative effects.

At-home monitoring and adjustments

- Monitor your progress by tracking key metrics such as food intake using **Cronometer, ketone levels** (0.5 mmol/l or more) using a blood meter, and **second morning urine pH** (6.5-7.0) using an electronic pH meter.
- Adjust your vegetable, magnesium citrate, and sodium bicarbonate intake as needed to **reach the desired urine pH level**.
- Regularly re-test until you can **predict results**.
- Listen to your body; if you experience adverse effects, **modify your diet** accordingly.

Exercise

- Work towards a **high VO$_2$ max** (see page 20). Studies show intermittent fasting is vastly more effective for individuals in the **top 25% of their age group**.
- **1 x HIRT weight training** per week, fasted.
- 1-2 x MAF HR cardio per week, fed or fasted

II. Additional resources

You can find most of the supplements, measuring devices, products and services that I mentioned in this book on the resource website I set up for readers of this book at: ReversingPKD.com/resources.

If you feel like you need a personalized approach and want to talk through your lab results, personal routines and food choices, you can reach out via ReversingPKD.com and book a free 15-minute consultation to see if I can help you further to reverse PKD.

III. FAQs

Why do only some patients have kidney pain?

Many PKD patients experience pain in their kidney area that can range from annoying to debilitating. Of course, the use of pain medication is a big problem (see page 194 on medications), as many PKD patients rely on them on a regular basis just to make it through the day. Many patients believe that their pain is caused by the structural pressure on parts of the kidneys or the interior of the bowels. While this can happen, in many cases this is not the main issue. We don't know for sure why some people experience more pain than others, as pain is not usually correlated with kidney or cyst size.

However, many reports from PKD patients who started on this program confirm that this is an issue that can resolve within a matter of weeks, even before any actual changes in size of the kidney or cysts become apparent on imaging. This leads us to the understanding that the pain experienced by some PKD patients is related to inflammation, and not necessarily structural pressure.

So if you are experiencing kidney pain, get started right away and curb the inflammation with this program.

Why are urinary tract infections common in PKD?

First off, the people with the worst cases of PKD are usually also the people with the worst blood sugar control, e.g. diabetics and prediabetic people. This is because sugar feeds cyst growth, as we have discussed before, but additionally in diabetics sugar begins to be excreted through the urine, which actually makes it sweet. This is by the way how it used to be diagnosed – by taste!

Now sweet urine of course also feeds bacteria. The more sugar in urine, the more likely you will get bacterial overgrowth in the bladder. When you stop the sugar and begin on a ketogenic diet, the sweet urine will soon become just regular urine and bacteria will like it less; but of course that's not enough.

As we discussed before, gram-negative bacteria seem to be a big issue as their endotoxins might well play a big role in the pathogenesis of PKD. Because of the higher permeability of the gut lining, bacteria have an easier entry to the rest of the body and some of them can make it to the bladder. Translocation of gut bacteria to other organs is a real problem. So maybe an increased propensity to develop UTIs is a sign that your gut wall is especially permeable and it's about time to start working on improving those tight junctions.

If we assume that gram-negative bacteria play a big role in creating UTIs, of course it would make sense to change their environment, meaning the urine, so that it becomes less hospitable for them. One study found that gram-negative bacteria grew in slightly acidic urine (pH 6.3), while gram-positive bacteria preferred a more alkaline urinary environment (pH 6.7).[1] We already know it is vital to keep our second morning urine pH between 6.5 and 7, so this will be extra motivation for anyone who is experiencing UTIs on a regular basis.

Can surgery help?

Some patients decide to get some of their cysts aspirated – that is, getting the fluid removed from them. The cysts usually get refilled with foam to prevent new fluid build-up inside the cysts. If you are considering this, make sure to talk to your surgeon and make them aware of the cystogenic properties of the very cyst fluid that they are going to remove. Some research suggests that spillage of this fluid can lead to more cyst growth, so it is vital they understand this fact and make sure no fluid is left behind and everything is properly cleaned up.

Fasting, keto, OMAD: Is more really better?
Many people reading about the benefits of fasting for PKD assume that more must be better. If intermittent fasting is good, multiple-day water fasting must be great. If a 16-hour intermittent fast is good, a one-meal-a day strategy must be amazing. If six days of a ketogenic diet per week are good, ongoing keto must be the best. These assumptions are not correct. As with most good things, these too can be overdone.

Too much fasting, meaning water only for a whole day or more, will liberate stored toxins from fat cells and excrete them into the gut. The problem is then that, if you fast for this long, there is not enough movement in the gut, nor enough fecal matter, to push the toxins that the body is trying to get rid of out. The result is reabsorption and redistribution of these toxins throughout the body. (See Chapter 11 on water fasting and protein fasting for more details on this – page 131.)

'OMAD', or one-meal-per-day, has become a popular strategy in the online world and some PKD patients aware of the benefits of fasting have taken notice and are only consuming one meal a day. This meal is usually very high in calories and contains most nutrients needed for the day. However, the human body is not always capable of absorbing all the nutrients that it needs in one sitting. So a long-term OMAD strategy brings with it a high risk for nutrient deficiencies. This is why it is not recommended.

FAQs

Why do you recommend carb days?
With all the benefits of a ketogenic diet, why should you even interrupt it? Can't we just stay in ketosis forever and thereby reduce cyst growth even more? While this might seem like a sensible idea, it doesn't just risk hormonal issues, but can actually increase your blood sugar in the long term, giving you something that looks like prediabetes on a blood test. If you are considering a long-term ketogenic diet, check your blood sugar and thyroid- and sex hormone status regularly. (Refer to the section on hormone testing for more details – page 197.)

Will my kids get PKD?
As in most genetic diseases, heritability depends on your specific form of PKD and the genes of your partner. If you have ADPKD, there is about a 50% chance your child will be affected; in ARPKD, it's just a 25% chance. If you want to be certain your children are not affected, there is an option of choosing IVF (in-vitro fertilization) with Preimplantation Genetic Diagnosis. In some countries, this method can be used to select an embryo that has two copies of the healthy gene and therefore will not have PKD.

Can my children get on the PKDproof program?
Yes! Skipping bad foods on the PKDproof program, and specifically the Bulletproof Diet, is safe for all ages; however, children are developing and therefore should not be in ketosis for extended periods of time. Carbs are still needed for proper development. It makes sense to start them off with most days of the week being carb days and then gradually ramping up keto days when they approach adulthood. Keeping an eye on their ultrasounds and blood tests will also help a great deal in informing your decision as to when to transition them to mostly ketogenic eating.

Do I really need to eat that many vegetables?

There are several reasons why I recommend eating most of the bulk on your plate as non-starchy vegetables. One of them is that we need to manage our pH level responsibly. Protein and fat both are on the acidic end of the spectrum, so our bodies need ample veggies to offset this acidity. Sure, drinking lemon water or even taking a couple of tablespoons of apple cider vinegar or some magnesium citrate can help a lot with pH, but the main star of the show is food. And non-starchy vegetables are by far your highest source of alkalizing (pH-increasing) nutrients. Another reason is that vegetables nourish your gut bacteria and give them the fuel to produce butyrate, which is an anti-inflammatory fatty acid and an HDAC inhibitor that also has specific benefits in PKD (addressed earlier on page 24). The final (and my favorite) reason to consume lots of veggies is that they are the perfect carrier for fat. Its pretty easy to hide a couple of tablespoons of butter or MCT oil in your broccoli, which will then taste all the better.

Flavor is king. Nobody said you needed to eat those veggies plain and raw. Instead, making a delicious stir-fry with great tasting sauce, some hearty soup, a huge veggie omelet, or even just a colorful salad with lots of bulletproof vinaigrette and some good-quality beef slices, are the way to do it. Check out the following recipes or even pictures of my meals at ReversingPKD.com to get some inspiration.

IV. Recipes

Clean keto staples

Bulletproof coffee

Ingredients:
- 1 cup mold-free coffee
- 20 g grass-fed butter
- 18 g C8 MCT oil
- Optional: 5-15 g organic cocoa butter

Instructions:

1. Brew 1 cup of coffee.
2. Preheat blender.
3. Add butter and MCT oil, and cocoa butter if using, to the blender.
4. Add brewed coffee and blend on high for 30 seconds.

Super-quick meal template

This is for anyone who doesn't want to spend more time in the kitchen than absolutely necessary. Use this template with any kind of frozen protein and frozen vegetables. Mix different vegetables for more diverse nutrition. Best results as well as maximum time savings are achieved when using a halogen oven and dedicated electric steamer, but can also be done with a pot and some water, a metal sieve and a standard oven.

Ingredients:
- 300 g frozen cauliflower, green beans or broccoli, etc
- 1 frozen grass-fed beef burger patty or sockeye salmon fillet
- Salt

Instructions:

1. Add the frozen veggies to your steamer, steam for 15-20 minutes.
2. Add the frozen protein to your halogen oven or normal oven and add salt.
3. Bake for 15-20 minutes at 320°F or 160°C (longer in a standard oven).
4. Drizzle with some MCT oil and serve with mustard, mayo or guacamole.

Standard meals

Grass-fed beef stir-fry

Ingredients (serves 1)
- 2 tbsp grass-fed butter
- 1 leek or red onion
- 6-8 oz grass-fed ground/minced beef: 36-48 g protein
- 1-2 cups medium-sized pieces of steamed cauliflower
- 1 cup medium-sized slices of steamed carrots
- 1 tbsp MCT oil
- Seasoning: salt, oregano and cumin to taste

Instructions:

1. Heat the grass-fed butter in a skillet over a medium heat.
2. Add leek or onion and sauté for a couple of minutes.
3. Add the ground/minced beef, season with salt and cook until slightly browned.
4. Add the steamed cauliflower and carrots to the skillet and stir well to combine.
5. Drizzle with 1 tablespoon of MCT oil before serving.

Vegetable and egg tajine

Ingredients (serves 1)
- carrots, cauliflower, and bell peppers
- 6 pastured eggs: 36 g protein
- 100 g feta cheese: 14 g protein
- 1 tbsp MCT oil
- Seasoning: salt, cumin and coriander to taste

Instructions:

1. Preheat the oven to 320°F (160°C).
2. Steam or cook the vegetables lightly in butter, ghee or tallow/lard.
3. Place the cooked vegetables in a tajine or baking dish.
4. Crack the eggs over the vegetables and stir in crumbled feta cheese.
5. Season with salt, cumin, and coriander.
6. Bake in the preheated oven until the eggs are set, about 30-40 minutes.
7. Drizzle with 1 tablespoon of MCT oil.

Sockeye salmon salad bowl

Ingredients (serves 1)
- 6-8 oz smoked sockeye salmon or fresh salmon fillet: 360-480 kcal, 30-41 g protein
- Romaine lettuce
- 1 medium cucumber, sliced, pitted
- 1 medium carrot, shredded
- 1/2 avocado
- Simple vinaigrette (olive oil, apple cider vinegar, and mustard)

Instructions:

1. Preheat your oven to 160°C/320°F.
2. Cover the salmon fillet in butter and bake it for 15-20 minutes or until it is cooked to your liking. Alternatively, use smoked sockeye salmon.
3. In a large bowl, mix the leafy greens, carrot and sliced cucumber.
4. Place the cooked salmon on top of the salad.
5. Drizzle the salad with the simple vinaigrette and serve immediately.

Easy liver

Ingredients (serves 1)
- ½ small leek or onion, sliced
- Butter, tallow/beef dripping or ghee
- 150 g liver, (1 slice): 250 kcal, 39 g protein
- Optional: 1 apple, sliced

Instructions:

1. Cook the leeks or onions (and apple if on a carb day) in fat on a low heat.
2. Add the liver and cook on a medium heat until the inside is light pink.

Simple beef and veggie soup

Ingredients (serves 1)
- 4 tbsp ghee, butter or tallow/beef dripping
- 1 shallot, diced
- 2 leeks or red onions, sliced
- 1 clove garlic, minced
- 1 kg diced beef (goulash)
- 2 cups bone broth
- 2 bay leaves
- 1 cup carrots, sliced
- 2 tbsp collagen powder
- 1 cup green beans, trimmed
- 1 cup cauliflower florets
- 1 cup broccoli florets
- 2 tsp salt
- 2 tbsp MCT oil

Instructions:

1. Preheat the oven to 320°F or 160°C.
2. In a large ovenproof pot, heat the fat over a medium heat then add the leeks or onions, shallot and garlic, sautéing until they are slightly softened.
3. Increase the heat to medium-high and add the beef to the pot. Sauté until slightly browned on all sides. Season the beef with 2 tsp of salt during browning.
4. Pour in the bone broth and add the bay leaves and carrots to the pot.
5. In a separate cup, dissolve the collagen powder in cold water, then add to the pot. If necessary, add extra water until everything is submerged.
6. Place the pot in the preheated oven and cook for approximately 90 minutes, or until the meat is tender.
7. Once the meat is tender, add the remaining veggies (leek, green beans, cauliflower and broccoli) to the pot and cook for an additional 30 minutes.
8. Once the vegetables are tender, remove the pot from the oven and stir in the MCT oil.
9. Taste and adjust the seasoning, if necessary, before serving.

Carb-day meals

Sweet potato fries and lamb bowl

Ingredients (serves 1)
- 300 g sweet potato ~ 258 kcal, 6 g protein, 60 g carbs
- 160 g lamb (lean part, cooked) ~ 448 kcal, 40 g protein, 16 g fat
- Warm coconut oil or equivalent
- Salt to taste
- Optional: Fresh herbs like parsley or cilantro for garnish
- 1 tbsp MCT oil ~ 126 kcal, 14 g fat

Instructions:

1. Wash, peel, cut, oil and salt the sweet potato.
2. Bake the sweet potato pieces until fork-tender, about 30-45 minutes.
3. Season the lamb with salt.
4. Heat the coconut oil in a pan over a medium heat and cook the lamb to your desired doneness, approximately 3-4 minutes per side for medium-rare. Alternatively, bake the lamb, rubbed with softened butter and rosemary.
5. Serve the cooked lamb beside the baked sweet potato fries. Add mustard or MCT oil mayo if desired.
6. Drizzle with 1 tbsp of MCT oil

Totals:

832 kcal, 46 g protein, 60 g carbs, 30 g fat

Organic sockeye salmon and white rice bowl

Ingredients (serves 1)
- 160 g sockeye salmon (cooked): 368 kcal, 40 g protein (approx.), 14.4 g fat
- 200 g white rice (cooked, thoroughly rinsed organic): 220 kcal,

4 g protein, 48 g carbs
- 1 tbsp coconut aminos: 10 kcal, 2 g carbs
- 1 tbsp MCT oil: 126 kcal, 14 g fat
- Optional: Green onions and sesame seeds for garnish

Instructions:

1. Thoroughly rinse the organic white rice under cold water until the water runs clear to remove any excess starch and pesticides. Cook according to the package instructions.
2. While the rice is cooking, season the salmon with salt.
3. Cook the salmon in a non-stick pan over a medium heat until it reaches your desired level of doneness, usually about 3-4 minutes per side.
4. Once the salmon and rice are cooked, place the rice in a bowl, top it with the cooked salmon.
5. Drizzle with coconut aminos and MCT oil and garnish with green onions and sesame seeds if desired.

Totals:

724 kcal, 44 g protein (approx.), 50 g carbs, 28.4 g fat

Protein fasting meals

Quick Brussels sprouts soup

Ingredients (serves 1)
- 150 g Brussels sprouts
- 1 cup bone broth
- 1 tbsp C8 MCT oil

Instructions:

1. Wash and trim the Brussels sprouts; cut them in half.
2. In a medium pot, warm the bone broth to a simmer over a medium-high heat.
3. Add the Brussels sprouts to the broth; reduce the heat to medium and let them simmer for about 10-15 minutes or until they are tender.
4. Once the Brussels sprouts are tender, turn off the heat and carefully blend the soup using an immersion blender until it reaches your desired consistency. Alternatively, you can transfer the soup to a blender.
5. Drizzle the C8 MCT oil over the soup and stir well before serving.

Totals:
230 kcal, 13 g protein, 14 g carbs, 14 g fat

Creamy broccoli and leek soup

Ingredients (serves 1)
- 1 tbsp ghee
- 1 cup or 100 g leek, sliced
- 1 clove garlic, minced
- 240 ml bone broth
- 3/4 cup or 100 g broccoli florets
- 1/2 cup or 100 ml full-fat coconut milk

Instructions:

1. Heat the ghee over a medium heat. Add the leeks and sauté for 1-2 minutes until it starts to turn translucent.
2. Add garlic and cook for 1 minute or until fragrant.
3. Pour in the broth; add the broccoli florets and leek. Season with salt to taste. Bring to the boil, then lower the heat to simmer for 15 minutes or until the broccoli is fork-tender. Add water if necessary.
4. Add the coconut milk and allow it to fully warm – about 1 minute.
5. Transfer the mixture to a food processor and purée until smooth.
6. Top with some fresh basil.

Totals:

400 kcal, 14 g protein, 15 g carbs, 32 g fat

Desserts, treats and fat-bombs

Panna cotta

Ingredients (serves 4)
- 1 cup blueberries
- 4 cups full-fat coconut milk
- 4 tbsp xylitol or stevia, to taste
- 1 tbsp grass-fed gelatin
- 2 tsp vanilla powder
- 4 tbsp grass-fed unsalted butter
- 1 tbsp MCT oil
- ½ cup shredded coconut

Instructions:

1. Place blueberries in a deep dish.
2. Heat 1 cup coconut milk with xylitol and gelatin until dissolved.
3. Blend remaining coconut milk with vanilla, butter, and oil.
4. Add hot coconut milk mixture and shredded coconut to the blender, pulse until mixed.
5. Pour over blueberries and refrigerate for 1 hour to set.

Keto ice cream

Ingredients (serves 2-3)
- 4 whole pastured eggs
- 4 pastured egg yolks
- 2 tsp (10 g) vanilla powder
- 1 g vitamin C or 10 drops apple cider vinegar or lime juice
- 7 tbsp (100 g) grass-fed unsalted butter
- 7 tbsp (100 g) coconut oil
- 3 tbsp + 2 tsp (53 g) MCT oil

- 5½ tbsp (82 g) erythritol
- Optional: ¼ to ½ cup (30 to 60 g) chocolate powder
- ½ cup (120 ml) water or ice

Instructions:

1. Blend all the ingredients except the water or ice until creamy.
2. Add water or ice and blend until well mixed.
3. Pour into an ice cream maker and churn until it reaches the desired consistency.

Cauliflower pizza

Ingredients (serves 1)
- 1 medium cauliflower
- 2 eggs
- 1 tbsp oregano
- ¼ cup white almond or macadamia flour
- Butter (optional)
- Grass-fed cheese (if you are not casein or lactose sensitive)
- Organic tomato pureé from a jar or carton
- Organic toppings

Instructions:

1. Grate the cauliflower and cook on a low heat with some butter for 15 minutes, then wring out the water using a cheesecloth. Alternatively, use a juicer to juice the cauliflower, then discard the juice and use the pulp.
2. Mix the cauliflower, eggs, oregano and nut flour to form a dough.
3. Roll out on a baking sheet and bake for 15-20 minutes at 160°C (320°F). .

Whey protein balls

Ingredients (10-20 balls)
- 2 tbsp erythritol
- 2 tbsp water
- 1 cup shredded coconut
- 15 g collagen
- 30 g grass-fed whey
- Optional: 2 tsp organic cocoa powder
- Optional: butter/coconut oil (make it a fat-bomb)

Instructions:

1. Mix the erythritol with water and let it sit.
2. Combine the rest of the dry ingredients.
3. Add erythritol water and knead to form a block.
4. If you like, add 50-100 g butter to increase calories and fat.
5. Shape into 10-20 balls and refrigerate for 30 minutes.

Coconut cacao fat-bomb

Ingredients (8 mini-muffin-sized bombs)
- ½ cup coconut oil, melted
- ½ cup cacao powder
- 8 drops liquid stevia
- 2 tbsp cacao nibs, to garnish (optional)

Instructions:

1. Combine all the ingredients except the cacao nibs and mix well.
2. Pour the mixture into silicone molds of your choosing (mini muffin size or similar).
3. Sprinkle the mixture in the molds with the cacao nibs.
4. Place the molds in the freezer until set.

Condiments and basic ingredients

Guacamole

Ingredients (serves 1-2)
- 1 avocado
- 2 tbsp MCT oil
- 2 tbsp apple cider vinegar
- 1 garlic clove, mashed
- 2 pinches sea salt
- 2 pinches oregano

Instructions:

1. Mash all the ingredients together on a plate using a potato masher until well combined.

Simple vinaigrette dressing

Ingredients (for one medium salad)
- 25 ml MCT oil or extra-virgin organic olive oil
- 25 ml apple cider vinegar
- 1 tsp mustard
- Salt
- Oregano
- Optional: 1 tsp erythritol

Instructions:

1. Combine all the ingredients in a salad-dressing shaker.
2. Shake well before serving.

MCT-oil mayo

Ingredients (to make about 210 ml mayo)
- 1 egg
- 150 ml MCT oil
- 1 pinch salt
- 1 tsp medium-hot mustard
- ¼ lemon, juiced

Instructions:

1. Place all the ingredients in a container.
2. Use an immersion blender, starting at the bottom and slowly moving upward over 10-20 seconds until the mixture thickens.
3. Taste and adjust the seasoning if needed.

Grass-fed beef bone broth

Ingredients
- 2 lb (0.9 kilos) grass-fed beef bones
- 3-4 l water
- 1 tbsp apple cider vinegar
- 1 leek or 2 onions, roughly diced
- 2 carrots, chopped
- 2 garlic cloves, smashed
- 2-4 tsp salt

Instructions:

1. Place the beef bones in an 8-liter slow cooker or a large pot.
2. Add 3-4 l water to cover the bones.
3. Add the apple cider vinegar, leeks or onions, carrots, and garlic cloves.
4. Sprinkle with salt, adjusting to your taste.
5. For slow cooker: Set to 'auto' (approximately 85°C/185°F) and simmer for 24 hours.

6. For stove top: Bring to a gentle boil, then simmer for a minimum of 2 hours; longer is better for a richer broth.
7. Strain the broth using a large sieve, optionally through a cloth for a clearer consistency.
8. Divide into 1-liter bags or 500-ml jars and freeze for later use.

Simple clean protein shake recipe

Ingredients (for one shake)
- 30 g pure grass-fed whey protein concentrate powder
- 10 g grass-fed collagen powder
- 1-2 tsp organic pure cocoa powder
- Stevia drops with vanilla flavor
- 18 g C8 MCT oil
- 1 cup water/coconut milk/grass-fed raw milk if tolerated

Instructions:

1. Get a steel shaker ball and a glass mason jar or similar and take that with you.
2. You can also add some protease enzymes to this shake to make it more digestible. Just make sure you let it sit for at least 30 minutes at room temperature.
3. Drink this slowly as liquid protein like this can be a bit difficult for some of us. If you get any pain or foamy urine, drink it more slowly the next time around or just use food.

Autophagy tea

Courtesy of Dr Joseph Mercola

Ingredients (makes 1 cup):
- 1 tsp pau d'arco powdered tea
- ½ tsp hydroxycitrate and garcinia (HCA/garcinia powder)

- ½ tsp quercetin powder
- ½ tsp glycine powder
- ½ tsp chamomile powder
- Lakanto monk fruit sweetener to taste (optional)

Instructions:

1. Add everything to a cup of water or chamomile tea.
2. Pro tip: You can just add all the ingredients in these ratios to a big mason jar and store the ready-made mix. Therefore, you will only have to go into your kitchen at night and take one big tablespoon of your premade powder, stir in some water or chamomile tea and drink it before bed. As a nice side effect, chamomile tea is very soothing.

If you are not going to go the tea route, you can always use the capsule forms of the ingredients. And if you're not going to buy all of them, I recommend starting with quercetin; 1000 mg should be a good starting dose.

High-absorption curcumin aka 'black sludge'

You can make a highly water-soluble curcumin supplement yourself if you want to save some money over the long term. There is a video on how to do it on my YouTube channel, but here is the basic recipe, courtesy of the chemist Brad Culkin, PhD, who open-sourced this recipe for the greater good. Be advised that this is an advanced recipe and needs to be followed with care.

Ingredients for 100 'size 000' capsules:
- 50 g food-grade sodium carbonate (not sodium bicarbonate)
- 15 g 95% curcuminoid powder
- 70 g food-grade vegetable glycerin

- 100 HPMC-coated capsules 'size 000'

Instructions:

1. Put on an FFP2 face mask and some goggles, as the steam of sodium carbonate is irritating to the eyes and lungs. Open windows.
2. Mix the sodium carbonate with the curcuminoid powder, heat the glycerin in a bain-marie-style water bath and slowly stir in tablespoon after tablespoon of the powder mix until it's all mixed in over 5-10 minutes. Heat just enough so the water does not bubble. I use a hand-held food mixer on a slow setting to continuously stir the mixture. Don't go too fast or it might thicken too much.
3. When you feel everything has incorporated well, dip a butter knife into the now deep-red mixture and swirl it around a glass of water. If you are seeing tiny orange particles floating on top of the water after everything has been stirred off of the butter knife, it hasn't dissolved fully yet. If after repeated tries you are still getting orange pieces floating on top, you might have to add more glycerin or sodium carbonate. You're looking for deep-red transparent water with no orange particles floating on top when you are doing the butter knife test.
4. When the butter knife test has been successful, you can now use a big 100-ml syringe to suck in some of the mixture and squirt it into each 'size 000' capsule. Time is of the essence as the mixture can thicken quite quickly. If it does, filtered water can be added to dilute it a bit. When you are done, close up the capsules and refrigerate. That's it.
5. Consume swiftly. (The shelf life of glycerin is 24 months.)

This is a very involved process and it might be too much for many readers but now you know there is a budget-friendly option to this more expensive supplement on my list. This way is almost 16 times cheaper than buying the ready-made capsules and yields about 160 mg of curcuminoids per capsule, so one of these per day is likely to be more than enough.

Personal care recipes

Homemade deodorant for light days

Ingredients
- 70 ml water
- 1 tsp baking soda

Instructions:

1. Combine the water and baking soda in a 500-ml glass beaker or jar with a pouring spout.
2. Stir the mixture continuously or shake well for about 5 minutes to ensure the baking soda is completely dissolved. This helps to prevent clogging the spray bottle.
3. Carefully pour the dissolved mixture into a spray bottle for future use.

Jojoba-based skin serum

Ingredients
- 40 ml organic jojoba oil
- 6 drops organic lavender essential oil
- 3 drops organic oregano essential oil
- 3 drops organic palmarosa essential oil
- 4 drops organic turmeric essential oil
- 3 drops organic juniper essential oil
- 2 drops organic lemon essential oil
- 1 drop of organic patchouli essential oil

Instructions:

1. Pour the jojoba oil into a 500-ml glass beaker or jar with a pouring spout.
2. Add the essential oils into the jojoba oil.
3. Swish the beaker gently to integrate all the essential oils with the jojoba oil.
4. Once fully combined, transfer the serum into a dark dropper bottle.
5. Use 10-15 drops on face in mornings.

References

Introduction

1. Torres JA, Kruger SL, Broderick C, Amarlkhagva T, Agrawal S, Dodam JR, Mrug M, Lyons LA, Weimbs T. Ketosis Ameliorates Renal Cyst Growth in Polycystic Kidney Disease. *Cell Metab* 2019; 30(6): 1007-1023.e5. doi: 10.1016/j.cmet.2019.09.012. PMID: 31631001; PMCID: PMC6904245.

Chapter 1: What is PKD?

1. Li SR, Gulieva RE, Helms L, Cruz NM, Vincent T, Fu H, Himmelfarb J, Freedman BS. Glucose absorption drives cystogenesis in a human organoid-on-chip model of polycystic kidney disease. *Nat Commun* 2022; 13(1): 7918.
doi: 10.1038/s41467-022-35537-2. PMID: 36564419.

Chapter 2: Basic molecular mechanisms of PKD

1. Lanktree MB, Haghighi A, Guiard E, et al. Prevalence Estimates of Polycystic Kidney and Liver Disease by Population Sequencing. *J Am Soc Nephrol* 2018; 29(10): 2593-2600. doi: 10.1681/ASN.2018050493. PMID: 30135240; PMCID: PMC6171271

2. Zhang Z, et al. Detection of PKD1 and PKD2 Somatic Variants in Autosomal Dominant Polycystic Kidney Cyst Epithelial Cells by Whole-Genome Sequencing. *J Am Soc Nephrol* 2021; 32(12): 3114-3129.

3. Dethlefsen MM, Bertholdt L, Gudiksen A, Stankiewicz T, Bangsbo J, van Hall G, Plomgaard P, Pilegaard H. Training state and skeletal muscle autophagy in response to 36 h of fasting. *J Appl Physiol* 2018; 125(5): 1609-1619.
doi: 10.1152/japplphysiol.01146.2017. PMID: 30161009.

4. Homer B. VO2 Max Essentials Part IV: Field tests for estimating VO2 max. www.physiologicallyspeaking.com 7 June 2023 https://bradyholmer.substack.com/p/vo2-max-essentials-part-4-field-tests (Accessed 19 Feb 2024)

5. Bellamy E. Exogenous ketones comparison (Ketone esters, ketone salts and C8 MCT oil) – experiment results. Ketosource 24 January 2019. https://web.archive.org/web/20221210012958/https://ketosource.co/exogenous-ketones-comparison/ (Accessed 19 Feb 2024)

6. Torres JA, Kruger SL, Broderick C, Amarlkhagva T, Agrawal S, Dodam JR, Mrug M, Lyons LA, Weimbs T. Ketosis Ameliorates Renal Cyst Growth in Polycystic Kidney Disease. *Cell Metab* 2019; 30(6): 1007-1023.e5. doi: 10.1016/j.cmet.2019.09.012. PMID: 31631001; PMCID: PMC6904245.

7. Seyfried TN, Yu G, Maroon JC, D'Agostino DP. Press-pulse: a novel therapeutic strategy for the metabolic management of cancer. *Nutr Metab (Lond)* 2017; 14: 19.
doi: 10.1186/s12986-017-0178-2. PMID: 28250801.

8. Podrini C, Rowe I, Pagliarini R, Costa ASH, et al. Dissection of metabolic reprogramming in polycystic kidney disease reveals coordinated rewiring of bioenergetic pathways. *Commun Biol* 2018; 1: 194. doi: 10.1038/s42003-018-0200-x. PMID: 30480096.

9. Kaminsky LA, Arena R, Myers J. Reference Standards for Cardiorespiratory Fitness Measured With Cardiopulmonary Exercise Testing: Data From the Fitness Registry and the Importance of Exercise National Database. *Mayo Clin Proc* 2015; 90(11): 1515-1523. doi: 10.1016/j.mayocp.2015.07.026. PMID: 26455884; PMCID: PMC4919021.

10. Kusumawati M, Abidin D, Darmawan A, Ruswadi S. The Influence of an 8-Week High-Intensity Interval Training Toward VO2Max. From the International Conference on Sport Science, Health and Physical Education (ICSSHPE 2019). *Advances in Health Sicence Research* 2020; 21: 216-219.

doi: 10.2991/ahsr.k.200214.058

11. Erlangga Z, Ghashang SK, Hamdan I, Melk A, et al. The effect of prolonged intermittent fasting on autophagy, inflammasome and senescence genes expressions: An exploratory study in healthy young males. *Human Nutrition & Metabolism* 2023; 32: 200189. doi: 10.1016/j.hnm.2023.200189.

12. Wang Y, Xu Y, Wu Y, Mahmood T, Chen J, Guo X, Wu W, Wang B, Guo Y, Yuan J. Impact of Different Durations of Fasting on Intestinal Autophagy and Serum Metabolome in Broiler Chicken. Animals (Basel). 2021 Jul 23;11(8):2183. doi: 10.3390/ani11082183. PMID: 34438641; PMCID: PMC8388447.

13. Zhou X, Fan LX, Sweeney WE Jr, Denu JM, Avner ED, Li X. Sirtuin 1 inhibition delays cyst formation in autosomal-dominant polycystic kidney disease. *J Clin Invest* 2013; 123(7): 3084-3098. doi: 10.1172/JCI64401. PMID: 23778143; PMCID: PMC4101988.

14. Lifespan News – Update on Resveratrol Controversy. Lifespan.io 7 March 2022. www.lifespan.io/news/lifespan-news-update-on-resveratrol-controversy/ (accessed 25 October 2023)

15. Li X. Epigenetics and autosomal dominant polycystic kidney disease. *Biochim Biophys Acta* 2011; 1812(10): 1213-1218. doi: 10.1016/j.bbadis.2010.10.008. PMID: 20970496; PMCID: PMC3413450.

16. Xia S, Li X, Johnson T, Seidel C, Wallace DP, Li R. Polycystin-dependent fluid flow sensing targets histone deacetylase 5 to prevent the development of renal cysts. *Development* 2010; 137(7): 1075-1084.
doi: 10.1242/dev.049437. PMID: 20181743; PMCID: PMC2835323.

Chapter 3: Looking deeper – The X factor

1. Offer DEMY, Woodhouse MA, 1970 Toxic metabolic defect in polycystic disease of kidney. Evidence from microscope studies. *Lancet* 1(7646): 547-50.

2. Yamaguchi, T., et al. Cyst fluid from a murine model of polycystic kidney disease stimulates fluid secretion, cyclic adenosine monophosphate accumulation, and cell proliferation by Madin-Darby canine kidney cells in vitro. *Am J Kidney Dis* 1995; 25(3): 471-477.

3. Grantham JJ, et al. Evidence for a potent lipid secretagogue in the cyst fluids of patients with autosomal dominant polycystic kidney disease. *J Am Soc Nephrol* 1995; 6(4): 1242-1249.

4. Avner ED, et al. Regression of genetically determined polycystic kidney disease in murine organ culture. *Experientia* 1986; 42(1): 77-80.

5. Miller-Hjelle MA, et al. Polycystic kidney disease: an unrecognized emerging infectious disease? *Emerg Infect Dis* 1997; 3(2): 113-127.

6. Gardner KD, Reed WP, Evan AP, et al. Endotoxin provocation of experimental renal cystic disease. *Kidney Int* 1987; 32(3): 329-334. doi: 10.1038/ki.1987.213

7. Miller MA, Prior RB, Horvath FJ, Hjelle JT. Detection of endotoxiuria in polycystic kidney disease patients by the use of the Limulus amebocyte lysate assay. *Am J Kidney Disease* 1990; 15(2): 117-122. doi: 10.1016/s0272-6386(12)80508-7.

8. Tremellen K, Pearce K. Dysbiosis of Gut Microbiota (DOGMA)- -a novel theory for the development of Polycystic Ovarian Syndrome. *Med Hypotheses* 2012; 79(1): 104-112.

9. Trott JF, Hwang VJ, Ishimaru T, et al. Arginine reprogramming in ADPKD results in arginine-dependent cystogenesis. *Am J Physiol Renal Physiol* 2018; 315(6): F1855-F1868. doi: 10.1152/ajprenal.00025.2018.

10. Gardner KD, Jr, Evan AP, Reed WP. Accelerated renal cyst development in deconditioned germ-free rats. *Kidney Int* 1986; 29(6):1116-1123.

11. Nolan JP. The role of intestinal endotoxin in liver injury: a long and evolving history. Hepatology 2010; 52(5): 1829-1835.

12. Meghji S, Qureshi W, Henderson B, Harris M. The role of endotoxin and cytokines in the pathogenesis of odontogenic cysts. *Arch Oral Biol* 1996; 41(6): 523-531. doi: 10.1016/0003-9969(96)00032-5

13. Neudorf H, Durrer C, Myette-Cote E, et al. Oral Ketone Supplementation Acutely Increases Markers of NLRP3 Inflammasome Activation in Human Monocytes. *Mol Nutr Food Res* 2019; 63(11): e1801171. doi: 10.1002/mnfr.201801171

Chapter 4: The template for the PKDproof program

1 Stallings VA, Adgent MA, Umbach DA, Zemel BS, et al. Soy-Based Infant Formula Feeding and Impact on Estrogen-Responsive Tissue. *FASEB Journal* 2017; 31: 958.2-958.2. doi: 10.1096/fasebj.31.1_supplement.958.2

2. Berndt WO, Hayes AW, Phillips RD. Effects of mycotoxins on renal function: mycotoxic nephropathy. *Kidney Int* 1980; 18(5): 656-664. doi: 10.1038/ki.1980.183. PMID: 7463958.

3. Sauer LA, Blask DE, Dauchy RT. Dietary factors and growth and metabolism in experimental tumors. *J Nutr Biochem*. 2007 Oct;18(10):637-49. doi: 10.1016/j.jnutbio.2006.12.009. PMID: 17418560.

4. Menezes LF, Lin CC, Zhou F, Germino GG. Fatty Acid Oxidation is Impaired in An Orthologous Mouse Model of Autosomal Dominant Polycystic Kidney Disease. *EBioMedicine* 2016 5: 183-92. doi: 10.1016/j.ebiom.2016.01.027. PMID: 27077126; PMCID: PMC4816756.

5. Jin R, Hao J, Yi Y, Yin D, et al. Dietary Fats High in Linoleic Acids Impair Antitumor T-cell Responses by Inducing E-FABP-Mediated Mitochondrial Dysfunction. *Cancer Res* 2021; 81(20): 5296-5310. doi: 10.1158/0008-5472.CAN-21-0757. PMID: 34400394; PMCID: PMC8530923.

6. Cassina L, Chiaravalli M, Boletta A. Increased mitochondrial fragmentation in polycystic kidney disease acts as a modifier of disease progression. *FASEB J* 2020; 34(5):6493-6507. doi: 10.1096/fj.201901739RR. Epub 2020 Apr 2. PMID: 32239723.

7. Senyilmaz-Tiebe D, Pfaff DH, Virtue S, Schwarz KV, et al. Dietary stearic acid regulates mitochondria in vivo in humans. *Nat Commun* 2018; 9(1): 3129. doi: 10.1038/s41467-018-05614-6. PMID: 30087348

8. Plourde M, Cunnane SC. Extremely limited synthesis of long chain polyunsaturates in adults: implications for their dietary essentiality and use as supplements. *Appl Physiol Nutr Metab* 2007; 32(4): 619-634. doi: 10.1139/H07-034. Erratum in: Appl Physiol *Nutr Metab* 2008; 33(1): 228-229. PMID: 17622276

Chapter 5: How to do the PKDproof program right

1. Pollack. *The Fourth Phase of Water: Beyond solid, liquid and vapor.* Ebner & Sons; 2013.
2. Howard M, Howard G, Orrego D. Resolving Pulmonary Artery Intimal Sarcoma via the Standard of Care combined with Metabolic Therapies. Version 3.5: 27 August 2023. Retrieved from https://www.youtube.com/watch?v=pm2ia_Nsfc8 11 May 2024.
3. Satirapoj B, Vongwattana P, Supasyndh O. Very low protein diet plus ketoacid analogs of essential amino acids supplement to retard chronic kidney disease progression. *Kidney Res Clin Pract* 2018; 37(4): 384-392. doi: 10.23876/j.krcp.18.0055
4. Hahn D, Hodson EM, Fouque D. Low protein diets for non-diabetic adults with chronic kidney disease. *Cochrane Database Syst Rev* 2020; 10(10): CD001892. doi: 10.1002/14651858.CD001892.pub5. PMID: 33118160
5. Obeid W, Hiremath S, Topf JM. Protein Restriction for CKD: Time to Move On. *Kidney360* 2022; 3(9): 1611-1615. doi: 10.34067/KID.0001002022. PMID: 36245656
6. Zamami R, Kohagura K, Kinjyo K, et al. The Association between Glomerular Diameter and Secondary Focal Segmental Glomerulosclerosis in Chronic Kidney Disease. *Kidney Blood Press Res* 2021; 46(4): 433-440. doi: 10.1159/000515528. PMID: 34315152
7. Kontessis P, Jones S, Dodds R, et al. Renal, metabolic and hormonal responses to ingestion of animal and vegetable proteins. *Kidney Int* 1990; 38(1): 136-144. doi: 10.1038/ki.1990.178
8. Phillips SM, Van Loon LJ. Dietary protein for athletes: from requirements to optimum adaptation. *J Sports Sci* 2011; 29 Suppl 1: S29-S38. doi: 10.1080/02640414.2011.619204. PMID: 22150425
9. Bellarby J, Tirado R, Leip A, Weiss F, Lesschen JP, Smith P. Livestock greenhouse gas emissions and mitigation potential in Europe. *Glob Chang Biol* 2013; 19(1): 3-18. doi: 10.1111/j.1365-2486.2012.02786.x. PMID: 23504717.
10. Salatin J. TEDx Talks: Cows, Carbon and Climate. TEDxCharlottesville [Video]. YouTube 14 January 2016. www.youtube.com/watch?v=exampleURL
11. Liu CM, Stegger M, Aziz M, et al. Escherichia coli ST131-H22 as a

Foodborne Uropathogen. *mBio* 2018; 9(4): e00470-18.
doi: 10.1128/mBio.00470-18. PMID: 30154256

12. EWG (Environmental Working Group. (2003). PCBs in Farmed
Salmon. Environmental Working Group 312 July 2003.
www.ewg.org/research/pcbs-farmed-salmon (Accessed 20 Feb
2024)

13. Mazi TA, Stanhope KL. Elevated Erythritol: A Marker of
Metabolic Dysregulation or Contributor to the Pathogenesis of
Cardiometabolic Disease? *Nutrients* 2023; 15(18): 4011.
doi: 10.3390/nu15184011. PMID: 37764794

14. Torres VE, Chapman AB, Devuyst O, Gansevoort RT, et al. TEMPO
3:4 Trial Investigators. Tolvaptan in patients with autosomal
dominant polycystic kidney disease. *N Engl J Med* 2012; 367(25):
2407-2418. doi: 10.1056/NEJMoa1205511. PMID: 23121377;
PMCID: PMC3760207.

15. Spital A. Tolvaptan in Autosomal Dominant Polycystic Kidney
Disease. [Letter to the Editor]. The New England Journal of
Medicine 2012. Retrieved from https://www.nejm.org/doi/
full/10.1056/NEJMoa1205511#article_letters

16. Rangan GK, Wong ATY, Munt A, et al. Prescribed Water Intake in
Autosomal Dominant Polycystic Kidney Disease. *NEJM Evidence*
2022; 1(1): EVIDoa2100021. doi: 10.1056/EVIDoa2100021

17. Dev H, Zhu C, Barash I, Blumenfeld JD, et al. Feasibility of Water
Therapy for Slowing Autosomal Dominant Polycystic Kidney
Disease Progression. *Kidney360* 2024 Apr 1.
doi: 10.34067/KID.0000000000000428. Epub ahead of print.
PMID: 38556640.

Chapter 6: Adjustments for low kidney function

1. Jing S-B, Li L, Ji D, et al. Effect of Chitosan on Renal Function in
Patients with Chronic Renal Failure. *Journal of Pharmacy and
Pharmacology* 1997; 49(7): 721–723. doi: 10.1111/j.2042-7158.1997.
tb06099.x

2. Schlesinger N. Dietary factors and hyperuricaemia. *Curr Pharm Des*
2005; 11(32): 4133-4138.
doi: 10.2174/138161205774913273. PMID: 16375734.

3. Kedar E, Simkin PA. A perspective on diet and gout. *Adv Chronic*

Kidney Dis 2012; 19(6): 392-397.
doi: 10.1053/j.ackd.2012.07.011. PMID: 23089274.]

4. Hassan W, Shrestha P, Sumida K, et al. Association of Uric Acid–Lowering Therapy With Incident Chronic Kidney Disease. *JAMA Netw Open* 2022; 5(6): e2215878.
doi:10.1001/jamanetworkopen.2022.15878]

5. Yang Y, Zhou Y, Cheng S, Sun JL, Yao H, Ma L. Effect of uric acid on mitochondrial function and oxidative stress in hepatocytes. *Genet Mol Res* 2016; 15(2). doi: 10.4238/gmr.15028644. PMID: 27420973.]

6. Qi X, Guan K, Liu C, Chen H, Ma Y, Wang R. Whey protein peptides PEW and LLW synergistically ameliorate hyperuricemia and modulate gut microbiota in potassium oxonate and hypoxanthine-induced hyperuricemic rats. *J Dairy Sci* 2023; 106(11): 7367-7381.
doi: 10.3168/jds.2023-23369. PMID: 37562644.

7. Pingali U, et al. A randomized, double-blind, positive-controlled, prospective, dose-response clinical study to evaluate the efficacy and tolerability of an aqueous extract of *Terminalia bellerica* in lowering uric acid and creatinine levels in chronic kidney disease subjects with hyperuricemia. *BMC Complement Med Ther* 2020; 20(1): 281.

8. Jelkmann W, et al. Effects of antioxidant vitamins on renal and hepatic erythropoietin production. *Kidney Int* 1997; 51(2): 497-501.

9. Wagner GS, Tephly TR. A possible role of copper in the regulation of heme biosynthesis through ferrochelatase. *Adv Exp Med Biol* 1975; 58(00): 343-354.

Chapter 7: Weekly schedule – timing

1. Jo H, Cha B, Kim H, Brito S, Kwak BM, Kim ST, Bin BH, Lee MG. α-Pinene Enhances the Anticancer Activity of Natural Killer Cells via ERK/AKT Pathway. *Int J Mol Sci* 2021; 22(2): 656.
doi: 10.3390/ijms22020656. PMID: 33440866; PMCID: PMC7826552.

2. Zhao C, Cao Y, Zhang Z, Nie D, Li Y. Cinnamon and Eucalyptus Oils Suppress the Inflammation Induced by Lipopolysaccharide In Vivo. Molecules. 2021; 26(23): 7410.
doi: 10.3390/molecules26237410. PMID: 34885991; PMCID: PMC8659246.

3. Li Y, Fu X, Ma X, Geng S, et al. Intestinal Microbiome-Metabolome Responses to Essential Oils in Piglets. *Front Microbiol* 2018; 9: 1988. doi: 10.3389/fmicb.2018.01988. PMID: 30210470; PMCID: PMC6120982.

4. Davis SL. The least harm principle may require that humans consume a diet containing large herbivores, not a vegan diet. *Journal of Agricultural and Environmental Ethics* 2003; 16(4): 387-394. https://philpapers.org/rec/DAVTLH

5. How many die for your food. *Farming Truth.* https://farmingtruth. weebly.com/blog/how-many-die-for-your-food-calculating-the-death-toll-of-crop-production-vs-livestock-production

6. Srikanthan P, Karlamangla AS. Muscle mass index as a predictor of longevity in older adults. *Am J Med* 2014; 127(6): 547-553. doi: 10.1016/j.amjmed.2014.02.007. PMID: 24561114

7. Lucas PA, Meadows JH, Roberts DE, Coles GA.. The risks and benefits of a low protein-essential amino acid-keto acid diet. *Kidney Int* 1986; 29(5):995-1003. doi: 10.1038/ki.1986.99 PMID: 3723930

8. Houser J, Komarek J, Kostlanova N, Cioci G, et al. A Soluble Fucose-Specific Lectin from Aspergillus fumigatus Conidia - Structure, Specificity and Possible Role in Fungal Pathogenicity. *PLOS ONE* 2013; 8(12): e83077. doi: 10.1371/journal.pone.0083077

Chapter 8: Common myths

1. Girardat-Rotar L, Puhan MA, Braun J, Serra AL. Long-term effect of coffee consumption on autosomal dominant polycystic kidneys disease progression: results from the Suisse ADPKD, a Prospective Longitudinal Cohort Study. *J Nephrol* 2018; 31(1): 87-94. doi: 10.1007/s40620-017-0396-8. PMID: 28386880; PMCID: PMC5778163.

2. Martins ML, Martins HM, Gimeno A. Incidence of microflora and of ochratoxin A in green coffee beans (Coffea arabica). *Food Addit Contam* 2003; 20(12): 1127-1131. doi: 10.1080/02652030310001620405. PMID: 14726276.

3. Roddy E, Choi HK. Epidemiology of gout. *Rheum Dis Clin North Am* 2014; 40(2): 155-175. doi: 10.1016/j.rdc.2014.01.001. PMID: 24703341; PMCID: PMC4119792.

4. Lee JE, McLerran DF, Rolland B, Chen Y, et al. Meat intake and cause-specific mortality: a pooled analysis of Asian prospective cohort studies. *Am J Clin Nutr* 2013; 98(4): 1032-1041. doi: 10.3945/ajcn.113.062638. PMID: 23902788; PMCID: PMC3778858.

Chapter 9: Lifestyle strategies

1. Krappitz M, Gallagher AR, Fedeles S. Is it Time to Fold the Cysts Away? *Trends Mol Med* 2016; 22(12): 997-999. doi: 10.1016/j.molmed.2016.10.001. PMID: 27793600.
2. Glembotski CC. Endoplasmic reticulum stress in the heart. *Circ Res* 2007; 101(10): 975-984. doi: 10.1161/CIRCRESAHA.107.161273. PMID: 17991891
3. Pchelin P, Shkarupa D, Smetanina N, Grigorieva T, Lapshin R, Schelchkova N, Machneva T, Bavrina A. Red light photobiomodulation rescues murine brain mitochondrial respiration after acute hypobaric hypoxia. *J Photochem Photobiol B* 2023; 239: 112643. doi: 10.1016/j.jphotobiol.2022.112643. PMID: 36610350.
4. Austin E, Huang A, Wang JY, Cohen M, Heilman E, Maverakis E, Michl J, Jagdeo J. Red Light Phototherapy Using Light-Emitting Diodes Inhibits Melanoma Proliferation and Alters Tumor Microenvironments. *Front Oncol* 2022; 12: 928484. doi: 10.3389/fonc.2022.928484. PMID: 35847848; PMCID: PMC9278815.
5. Millet-Boureima C, Rozencwaig R, Polyak F, Gamberi C. Cyst Reduction by Melatonin in a Novel *Drosophila Model* of Polycystic Kidney Disease. *Molecules* 2020; 25(22): 5477. doi: 10.3390/molecules25225477. PMID: 33238462; PMCID: PMC7700119.
6. Arangino S, Cagnacci A, Angiolucci M, Vacca AM, Longu G, Volpe A, Melis GB. Effects of melatonin on vascular reactivity, catecholamine levels, and blood pressure in healthy men. *Am J Cardiol* 1999; 83(9): 1417-1419. doi: 10.1016/s0002-9149(99)00112-5. PMID: 10235107.

Chapter 10: Tracking your progress

1. Strubl S, et al. Ketogenic dietary interventions in autosomal dominant polycystic kidney disease-a retrospective case series study: first insights into feasibility, safety and effects. *Clin Kidney J* 2022; 15(6): 1079-1092.
2. Borsche L, Glauner B, von Mendel J. COVID-19 Mortality Risk Correlates Inversely with Vitamin D3 Status, and a Mortality Rate Close to Zero Could Theoretically Be Achieved at 50 ng/mL 25(OH)D3: Results of a Systematic Review and Meta-Analysis. *Nutrients* 2021; 13(10): 3596. doi: 10.3390/nu13103596. PMID: 34684596
3. Marshall RP, Droste JN, Giessing J, Kreider RB. Role of Creatine Supplementation in Conditions Involving Mitochondrial Dysfunction: A Narrative Review. *Nutrients* 2022; 14(3): 529. doi: 10.3390/nu14030529. PMID: 35276888
4. Robbins M. *Root Cause Protocol Blog.* https://therootcauseprotocol.com
5. Rind B (md). Thyroid scale overview. Retrieved from https://web.archive.org/web/20140702001329/ www.drrind.com/therapies/thyroid-scale#defining (Accessed 20 Feb 2024)

Chapter 11: What to do regularly

1. Mercola J. *Ketofast: Rejuvenate your health with a step-by-step guide to timing your ketogenic meals.* Hay House; 2021.
2. Mercola J. *The Ketofast Cookbook: Recipes for intermittent fasting and timed ketogenic meals.* Hay House; 2019.
3. Vendramini LC, Nishiura JL, Baxmann AC, Heilberg IP. Caffeine intake by patients with autosomal dominant polycystic kidney disease. *Braz J Med Biol Res.* 2012; 45(9):834-40. doi: 10.1590/s0100-879x2012007500120. PMID: 22801417.
4. Ito S. High-intensity interval training for health benefits and care of cardiac diseases - The key to an efficient exercise protocol. *World J Cardiol* 2019; 11(7): 171-188. doi: 10.4330/wjc.v11.i7.171. PMID: 31565193.
5. Francois ME, Little JP. Effectiveness and safety of high-intensity

interval training in patients with type 2 diabetes. *Diabetes Spectr* 2015; 28(1): 39-44. doi: 10.2337/diaspect.28.1.39. PMID: 25717277.

6. Creighton Personal Training. HIRT – A Safer, More Effective Alternative to HIIT. www.creightonpt.com/

7. Agostini D, Natalucci V, Baldelli G, De Santi M, et al. New Insights into the Role of Exercise in Inhibiting mTOR Signaling in Triple-Negative Breast Cancer. *Oxid Med Cell Longev* 2018; 2018: 5896786. doi: 10.1155/2018/5896786. PMID: 30363988; PMCID: PMC6186337.

8. Attia P, Attia P. (2022, 1. September). Peter Attia on Zone 2 and Zone 5 Training. Peter Attia. https://peterattiamd.com/exercising-for-longevity-peter-on-zone-2-and-zone-5-training/

9. Zhu Y , Teng T , Wang H , Guo H , et al . Quercetin inhibits renal cyst growth in vitro and via parenteral injection in a polycystic kidney disease mouse model. *Food Funct* 2018; 9(1):389-396. doi: 10.1039/c7fo01253e. PMID: 29215110.

10. Vicente-Vicente L, González-Calle D, Casanova AG, Hernández-Sánchez MT, et al. Promising Clinical Candidate for the Prevention of Contrast-Induced Nephropathy. *Int J Mol Sci* 2019; 20(19): 4961. doi: 10.3390/ijms20194961. PMID: 31597315.

11. Clifton PM. Effect of Grape Seed Extract and Quercetin on Cardiovascular and Endothelial Parameters in High-Risk Subjects. *J Biomed Biotechnol* 2004; 2004(5): 272-278. doi: 10.1155/S1110724304403088. PMID: 15577189

12. Lu NT, Crespi CM, Liu NM, Vu JQ, et al. A Phase I Dose Escalation Study Demonstrates Quercetin Safety and Explores Potential for Bioflavonoid Antivirals in Patients with Chronic Hepatitis C. *Phytother Res* 2016; 30(1): 160-1688. doi: 10.1002/ptr.5518. Epub 2015 Dec 1. PMID: 26621580; PMCID: PMC5590840.]

13. Stettner N, Rosen C, Bernshtein B, Gur-Cohen S, et al. Induction of Nitric-Oxide Metabolism in Enterocytes Alleviates Colitis and Inflammation-Associated Colon Cancer. *Cell Rep* 2018; 23(7): 1962-1976. doi: 10.1016/j.celrep.2018.04.053. PMID: 29768197; PMCID: PMC5976577

14. Reizine, F., Grégoire, M., Lesouhaitier, M., Coirier, V., et al. Beneficial effects of citrulline enteral administration on sepsis-induced T cell mitochondrial dysfunction. *Proceedings of the*

National Academy of Sciences of the United States of America 2022; 119. doi: 10.1073/pnas.2115139119.

15. Suzuki T, Morita M, Kobayashi Y, Kamimura A. Oral L-citrulline supplementation enhances cycling time trial performance in healthy trained men: Double-blind randomized placebo-controlled 2-way crossover study. *J Int Soc Sports Nutr* 2016; 13: 6. doi: 10.1186/s12970-016-0117-z. PMID: 26900386; PMCID: PMC4759860.

16. Papadia C, Osowska S, Cynober L, Forbes A. Citrulline in health and disease. Review on human studies. *Clin Nutr* 2018; 37(6 Pt A): 1823-1828. doi: 10.1016/j.clnu.2017.10.009. PMID: 29107336.

17. Romero MJ, Yao L, Sridhar S, Bhatta A, Dou H, Ramesh G, Brands MW, Pollock DM, Caldwell RB, Cederbaum SD, Head CA, Bagi Z, Lucas R, Caldwell RW. l-Citrulline Protects from Kidney Damage in Type 1 Diabetic Mice. *Front Immunol* 2013; 4: 480. doi: 10.3389/fimmu.2013.00480. PMID: 24400007; PMCID: PMC3871963.

18. McFarlin BK, Henning AL, Bowman EM, Gary MA, Carbajal KM. Oral spore-based probiotic supplementation was associated with reduced incidence of post-prandial dietary endotoxin, triglycerides, and disease risk biomarkers. *World J Gastrointest Pathophysiol* 2017; 8(3): 117-126. doi: 10.4291/wjgp.v8.i3.117. PMID: 28868181; PMCID: PMC5561432.

19. Shi-Bing Jing, Leishi Li, Daxi Ji, Yasuyuki Takiguchi, Tatsuaki Yamaguchi, Effect of Chitosan on Renal Function in Patients with Chronic Renal Failure. *Journal of Pharmacy and Pharmacology* 1997; 49(7): 721–723. doi: 10.1111/j.2042-7158.1997.tb06099.x

20. Takayama S, et al. 2021 Partially hydrolyzed guar gum attenuates non-alcoholic fatty liver disease in mice through the gut-liver axis. *World J Gastroenterol* 2021; 27(18): 2160-2176.

21. Wang Y, Xie Z, Zhang X, et al. Effect of Arabinogalactan on Intestinal Alkaline Phosphatase, Bacterial Endotoxin and Serum Cytokines in Type 2 Diabetic Rats[J]. *Science and Technology of Food Industry* 2021; 42(14): 334–340. (In Chinese with English abstract). doi: 10.13386/j.issn1002-0306.2020090167

22. Chen Q, Chen O, Martins IM, et al. Collagen peptides ameliorate intestinal epithelial barrier dysfunction in immunostimulatory Caco-2 cell monolayers via enhancing tight junctions. *Food Funct*

2017; 22;8(3): 1144-1151. doi: 10.1039/c6fo01347c. PMID: 28174772

23. McCarty MF, Lerner A. Perspective: Prospects for Nutraceutical Support of Intestinal Barrier Function. *Adv Nutr* 2021; 12(2): 316-324. doi: 10.1093/advances/nmaa139. PMID: 33126251

24. Toteda G, Vizza D, Lupinacci S, Perri A, Scalise MF, Indiveri C, Puoci F, Parisi OI, Lofaro D, La Russa A, Gigliotti P, Leone F, Pochini L, Bonofiglio R. Olive leaf extract counteracts cell proliferation and cyst growth in an in vitro model of autosomal dominant polycystic kidney disease. *Food Funct* 2018; 9(11):5925-5935. doi: 10.1039/c8fo01481g. PMID: 30375624.

25. Li Y, Gao J, Yang X, Li T, Yang B, Aili A. Combination of curcumin and ginkgolide B inhibits cystogenesis by regulating multiple signaling pathways. *Mol Med Rep* 2021; 23(3): 195. doi: 10.3892/mmr.2021.11834. PMID: 33495815

26. Gao J, Li Y, Wang X, Hao X, et al. The combination of curcumin and ginkgolide B reduces cyst growth by multiple cell signaling pathways (LB586). *FASEB Journal* 2014; 28: LB586. doi:10.1096/fasebj.28.1_supplement.lb586

27. Yuajit C, Chatsudthipong V. Nutraceutical for Autosomal Dominant Polycystic Kidney Disease Therapy. *J Med Assoc Thai* 2016; 99 Suppl 1: S97-103. PMID: 26817244.

28. Tayefi-Nasrabadi H, Sadigh-Eteghad S, Aghdam Z. The effects of the hydroalcohol extract of Rosa canina L. fruit on experimentally nephrolithiasic Wistar rats. *Phytother Res* 2012; 26(1): 78-85. doi: 10.1002/ptr.3519. PMID: 21544885

29. Walsh NP, Blannin AK, Robson PJ, et al. Glutamine, Exercise and Immune Function. *Sports Med* 1998; 26: 177–191. doi: 10.2165/00007256-199826030-00004

30. Darmaun D, Welch S, Rini A, Sager BK, Altomare A, Haymond MW. Phenylbutyrate-induced glutamine depletion in humans: effect on leucine metabolism. *Am J Physiol* 1998; 274(5): E801-7. doi: 10.1152/ajpendo.1998.274.5.E801. PMID: 9612237.3D.

31. Zhang G, Wang Y, Zhang Y, Wan X, et al. Anti-cancer activities of tea epigallocatechin-3-gallate in breast cancer patients under radiotherapy. *Curr Mol Med* 2012; 12(2): 163-76. doi: 10.2174/156652412798889063. PMID: 22280355.

32. Elsakka AMA, Bary MA, Abdelzaher E, Elnaggar M, Kalamian M, et al. Management of Glioblastoma Multiforme in a Patient

Treated with Ketogenic Metabolic Therapy and Modified Standard of Care: A 24-Month Follow-Up. *Front Nutr* 2018; 5: 20. doi: 10.3389/fnut.2018.00020. PMID: 29651419.

33. Zhang P, Wang Q, Lin Z, Yang P, et al. Berberine Inhibits Growth of Liver Cancer Cells by Suppressing Glutamine Uptake. *Onco Targets Ther* 2019; 12: 11751-11763. doi: 10.2147/OTT.S235667

34. Ozkurt S, Dogan I, Ozcan O, Fidan N, Bozaci I, Yilmaz B, Bilgin M. Correlation of serum galectin-3 level with renal volume and function in adult polycystic kidney disease. *Int Urol Nephrol* 2019; 51(7): 1191-1197.
    doi: 10.1007/s11255-019-02156-8. PMID: 31012038.

35. Sathisha UV, Jayaram S, Harish Nayaka MA, Dharmesh SM. Inhibition of galectin-3 mediated cellular interactions by pectic polysaccharides from dietary sources. *Glycoconj J* 2007; 24(8): 497-507. doi: 10.1007/s10719-007-9042-3. PMID: 17525829.

36. Lazebnik Y. Cell fusion as a link between the SARS-CoV-2 spike protein, COVID-19 complications, and vaccine side effects. *Oncotarget* 2021; 12(25): 2476-2488. doi: 10.18632/oncotarget.28088. PMID: 34917266; PMCID: PMC8664391.]

37. Kim ES, Jeon MT, Kim KS, Lee S, Kim S, Kim DG. Spike Proteins of SARS-CoV-2 Induce Pathological Changes in Molecular Delivery and Metabolic Function in the Brain Endothelial Cells. *Viruses* 2021; 13(10): 2021. doi: 10.3390/v13102021. PMID: 34696455; PMCID: PMC8538996.

38. BioNTech. (2020). A phase 1/2/3, placebo-controlled, randomized, observer-blind, dose-finding study to evaluate the safety, tolerability, immunogenicity, and efficacy of SARS-CoV-2 RNA vaccine candidates against COVID-19 in healthy individuals (Protocol No. C4591001).

39. Pfizer. p. 68 https://cdn.pfizer.com/pfizercom/2020-11/C4591001_Clinical_Protocol_Nov2020.pdf [original URL offline, archived here: https://archive.org/details/c-4591001-clinical-protocol-nov-2020-pfizer-bio-ntech_202107

40. Röltgen K. Nielsen SCA, Silva O, Younes SF, et al. Immune imprinting, breadth of variant recognition, and germinal center response in human SARS-CoV-2 infection and vaccination. *Cell* 2022; 185(6): 1025-1040.e14. doi: 10.1016/j.cell.2022.01.018. PMID: 35148837; PMCID: PMC8786601.

41. Mulroney TE, Pöyry T, Yam-Puc JC, et al. N1-methylpseudouridylation of mRNA causes +1 ribosomal frameshifting. *Nature* 2024; 625(7993): 189-194. doi: 10.1038/s41586-023-06800-3. PMID: 38057663

42. Hulscher N, Procter BC, Wynn C, McCullough PA. Clinical Approach to Post-acute Sequelae After COVID-19 Infection and Vaccination. *Cureus* 2023; 15(11): e49204. doi: 10.7759/cureus.49204. PMID: 38024037; PMCID: PMC10663976.

43. Parry PI, Lefringhausen A, Turni C, Neil CJ, et al. 'Spikeopathy': COVID-19 Spike Protein Is Pathogenic, from Both Virus and Vaccine mRNA. *Biomedicines* 2023; 11(8): 2287. doi: 10.3390/biomedicines11082287. PMID: 37626783

44. Seneff S, Nigh G, Kyriakopoulos AM, McCullough PA. Innate immune suppression by SARS-CoV-2 mRNA vaccinations: The role of G-quadruplexes, exosomes, and MicroRNAs. *Food Chem Toxicol* 2022; 164: 113008. doi: 10.1016/j.fct.2022.113008. PMID: 35436552

45. Environmental Health Trust, et al, Consolidated with Children's Health Defense, et al. Environmental Health Trust v. Federal Communications Commission (2021). No. 20-1025, 20-1138 (U.S. Ct. App. D.C. Cir. August 13, 2021) *Findlaw* https://caselaw.findlaw.com/court/us-dc-circuit/2141117.html (Accessed 20 Feb 2024)

46. Pall ML. Wi-Fi is an important threat to human health. *Environ Res* 2018; 164: 405-416. doi: 10.1016/j.envres.2018.01.035. PMID: 29573716.

47. Mercola J. *EMF*D: 5G, Wi-Fi and Cell Phones – Hidden harms and how to protect yourself.* Hay House; 2012.

48. Luo C, Yang C, Wang X, Chen Y, Liu X, Deng H. Nicotinamide reprograms adipose cellular metabolism and increases mitochondrial biogenesis to ameliorate obesity. *J Nutr Biochem* 2022; 107: 109056. doi: 10.1016/j.jnutbio.2022.109056. PMID: 35609856.

49. Kumar P, Liu C, Hsu JW, Chacko S, Minard C, Jahoor F, Sekhar RV. Glycine and N-acetylcysteine (GlyNAC) supplementation in older adults improves glutathione deficiency, oxidative stress, mitochondrial dysfunction, inflammation, insulin resistance,

endothelial dysfunction, genotoxicity, muscle strength, and cognition: Results of a pilot clinical trial. *Clin Transl Med* 2021; 11(3): e372. doi: 10.1002/ctm2.372. PMID: 33783984

50. de Paz-Lugo P, Lupiáñez JA, Meléndez-Hevia E. High glycine concentration increases collagen synthesis by articular chondrocytes in vitro: acute glycine deficiency could be an important cause of osteoarthritis. *Amino Acids* 2018; 50(10): 1357-1365. doi: 10.1007/s00726-018-2611-x. PMID: 30006659

51. Chen Q, Chen O, Martins IM, Hou H, Zhao X, Blumberg JB, Li B. Collagen peptides ameliorate intestinal epithelial barrier dysfunction in immunostimulatory Caco-2 cell monolayers via enhancing tight junctions. *Food Funct* 2017; 8(3): 1144-1151. doi: 10.1039/c6fo01347c. PMID: 28174772.

52. Cuñetti L, Manzo L, Peyraube R, Arnaiz J, Curi L, Orihuela S. Chronic Pain Treatment With Cannabidiol in Kidney Transplant Patients in Uruguay. *Transplant Proc* 2018; 50(2): 461-464. doi: 10.1016/j.transproceed.2017.12.042. PMID: 29579828.

53. Davis DR, Epp MD, Riordan HD. Changes in USDA food composition data for 43 garden crops, 1950 to 1999. *J Am Coll Nutr* 2004; 23(6): 669-82. doi: 10.1080/07315724.2004.10719409. PMID: 15637215

54. Scheer FA, Van Montfrans GA, van Someren EJ, Mairuhu G, Buijs RM. Daily nighttime melatonin reduces blood pressure in male patients with essential hypertension. *Hypertension* 2004; 43(2): 192-197. doi: 10.1161/01.HYP.0000113293.15186.3b. PMID: 14732734.

55. Scheer FA. Potential use of melatonin as adjunct antihypertensive therapy. *Am J Hypertens* 2005; 18(12 Pt 1): 1619-1620. doi: 10.1016/j.amjhyper.2005.07.013. PMID: 16364835.

56. Xu S, Li L, Wu J, An S, Fang H, Han Y, Huang Q, Chen Z, Zeng Z. Melatonin Attenuates Sepsis-Induced Small-Intestine Injury by Upregulating SIRT3-Mediated Oxidative-Stress Inhibition, Mitochondrial Protection, and Autophagy Induction. *Front Immunol* 2021; 12: 625627. doi: 10.3389/fimmu.2021.625627. PMID: 33790896; PMCID: PMC8006917.

57. Możdżan M, Możdżan M, Chałubiński M, Wojdan K, Broncel M. The effect of melatonin on circadian blood pressure in patients with type 2 diabetes and essential hypertension. *Arch Med Sci*

2014; 10(4):669-75. doi: 10.5114/aoms.2014.44858.
PMID: 25276149; PMCID: PMC4175768.]

58. Kim JY, Gum SN, Paik JK, Lim HH, et al. Effects of nattokinase on blood pressure: a randomized, controlled trial. *Hypertens Res* 2008; 31(8): 1583-1588. doi: 10.1291/hypres.31.1583. PMID: 18971533.

Chapter 12: Common pitfalls

1. Kephart WC, Mumford PW, Mao X, Romero MA, et al. The 1-Week and 8-Month Effects of a Ketogenic Diet or Ketone Salt Supplementation on Multi-Organ Markers of Oxidative Stress and Mitochondrial Function in Rats. *Nutrients* 2017; 9(9): 1019. doi: 10.3390/nu9091019. PMID: 28914762.

2. Howard M, Howard G, Orrego D. Resolving Pulmonary Artery Intimal Sarcoma via the Standard of Care combined with Metabolic Therapies. Version 3.5: 27 August 2023. Retrieved from https://www.youtube.com/watch?v=pm2ia_Nsfc8 11 May 2024.

Chapter 13: About common medications

1. Nagao S, Nishii K, Yoshihara D, et al. Calcium channel inhibition accelerates polycystic kidney disease progression in the Cy/+ rat. *Kidney Int* 2008; 73(3): 269-277.
doi: 10.1038/sj.ki.5002629. PMID: 17943077

2. Haider DG, Sauter T, Lindner G, Masghati S, et al. Use of calcium channel blockers is associated with mortality in patients with chronic kidney disease. *Kidney and Blood Pressure Research* 2015; 40(6): 630-638. doi: 10.1159/000368539

3. Stoschitzky K, Sakotnik A, Lercher P, Zweiker R, Maier R, Liebmann P, Lindner W. Influence of beta-blockers on melatonin release. *Eur J Clin Pharmacol* 1999; 55(2): 111-115.
doi: 10.1007/s002280050604. PMID: 10335905

4. Scheer FA, Morris CJ, Garcia JI, Smales C, Kelly EE, Marks J, Malhotra A, Shea SA. Repeated melatonin supplementation improves sleep in hypertensive patients treated with beta-blockers: a randomized controlled trial. *Sleep* 2012; 35(10): 1395-1402. doi: 10.5665/sleep.2122. PMID: 23024438; PMCID: PMC3443766.

5. Watanabe H, Martini AG, Brown EA, Liang X, Medrano S, Goto S, Narita I, Arend LJ, Sequeira-Lopez MLS, Gomez RA. Inhibition of the renin-angiotensin system causes concentric hypertrophy of renal arterioles in mice and humans. *JCI Insight* 2021; 6(24): e154337. doi: 10.1172/jci.insight.154337. PMID: 34762601; PMCID: PMC8783690.

6. Yamal J, Martinez J, Osani MC, Du XL, et al. Mortality and Morbidity Among Individuals with Hypertension Receiving a Diuretic, ACE Inhibitor, or Calcium Channel Blocker: A Secondary Analysis of a Randomized Clinical Trial. *JAMA Netw Open* 2023; 6(12): e2344998.
doi: 10.1001/jamanetworkopen.2023.44998

7. Zhou X, Davenport E, Ouyang J, Hoke ME, et al. Pooled Data Analysis of the Long-Term Treatment Effects of Tolvaptan in ADPKD. *Kidney Int Rep* 2022; 7(5): 1037-1048.
doi: 10.1016/j.ekir.2022.02.009. PMID: 35570988; PMCID: PMC9091612.

8. U.S. Food and Drug Administration. (2013, April 30). FDA Drug Safety Communication: FDA limits duration and usage of Samsca (tolvaptan) due to possible liver injury leading to organ transplant or death. Retrieved from www.fda.gov/drugs/drug-safety-and-availability/fda-drug-safety-communication-fda-limits-duration-and-usage-samsca-tolvaptan-due-possible-liver

9. Perneger TV, Whelton PK, Klag MJ. Risk of kidney failure associated with the use of acetaminophen, aspirin, and nonsteroidal antiinflammatory drugs. *N Engl J Med* 1994; 331(25): 1675-1679.
doi: 10.1056/NEJM199412223312502. PMID: 7969358.

10. Loomans-Kropp HA, Pinsky P, Cao Y, Chan AT, Umar A. Association of Aspirin Use With Mortality Risk Among Older Adult Participants in the Prostate, Lung, Colorectal, and Ovarian Cancer Screening Trial. *JAMA Netw Open* 2019; 2(12): e1916729. doi: 10.1001/jamanetworkopen.2019.16729. Erratum in: *JAMA Netw Open* 2020; 3(1): e1921081. PMID: 31800071; PMCID: PMC6902761.

11. Park A. Should You Take a Daily Aspirin to Prevent Heart Attacks or Strokes? *Time* 1 December 2016.
https://time.com/4586868/daily-aspirin-heart-attacks/ (Accessed 20 Feb 2024)

Chapter 14: Barriers to healing

1. Ross E. *The Paleo Thyroid Solution 2nd Edition*. Bradventures LLC; 2020.
2. Kalish D. The Kalish Method: Healing the Body, Mapping the Mind.
3. Brandão R, Santos FW, Zeni G, Rocha JB, Nogueira CW. DMPS and N-acetylcysteine induced renal toxicity in mice exposed to mercury. *Biometals* 2006; 19(4): 389-398. doi: 10.1007/s10534-005-4020-3. PMID: 16841248.
4. Zalups RK, Gelein RM, Cernichiari E. DMPS as a rescue agent for the nephropathy induced by mercuric chloride. *J Pharmacol Exp Ther* 1991; 256(1): 1-10. PMID: 1671092.
5. Nathan N. Toxic: Heal Your Body from Mold Toxicity, Lyme Disease, Multiple Chemical Sensitivities, and Chronic Environmental Illness. Victory Belt; 2018.
6. Levy TE. *Hidden Epidemic: Silent Oral Infections Cause Most Heart Attacks and Breast Cancers*. Medfox Publishing; 2017.

Appendices: III FAQs

1. Hattah DKA, Sjahril R, Sriwijaya S. The Turbidity, pH, Direct Gram as Predictors of Symptomatic Urinary Tract Infections in Pregnant Women. *Nusantara Medical Science Journal* 2022; 7(2): 98-105.

Index

Footnote: 'A' in brackets following a page number refers to items in the Appendix.

Footnote: 'A' in brackets following a page number refers to items in the Appendix.

Footnote: 'A' in brackets following a page number refers to items in the Appendix.

Index

Footnote: 'A' in brackets following a page number refers to items in the Appendix.

Footnote: 'A' in brackets following a page number refers to items in the Appendix.

Footnote: 'A' in brackets following a page number refers to items in the Appendix.

Also from Hammersmith Health Books...

ECOLOGICAL MEDICINE
The Antidote to Big Pharma and Fast Foods
SECOND EDITION

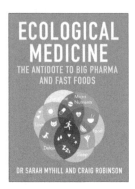

Launched originally in 2020, this latest edition is a distillation of over four decades of Dr Sarah Myhill's experiences as a doctor, starting out in the NHS and moving into independent practice to esape the straitjacket of official clinical guidelines. Writing with Craig Robinson, she clearly outlines the roadmap to recovery and illustrates this from the perspective of all medical diseases, from cancer and cardiology to neurology and nephrology. These medical 'ologies are further illustrated by real case histories that have been shaped, and continue to shape, her medical practice.

'Ecological Medicine is Sarah Myhill's magnum opus. As such it should be in every medical practice. It pulls no punches in looking at the degeneration of our health, overseen by doctors corrupted by Big Pharma. ... If you buy only one book from this whole field, this should be it.'

David Lorimer, Paradigm Explorer: Journal of the
Scientific and Medical Network